MRCS System Modules:

The Complete Test

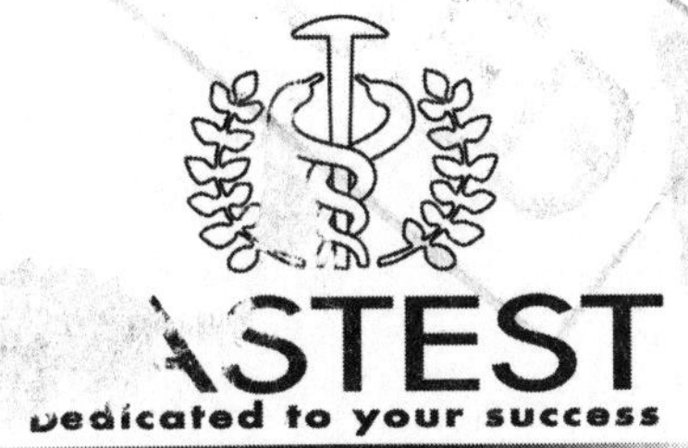

MRCS System Modules: The Complete Test

Christopher L H Chan
BSc (Hons) MBBS FRCS

Overseas Colorectal Surgical Fellow
Concord General Hospital
University of Sydney

SpR (General Surgery) SE Thames

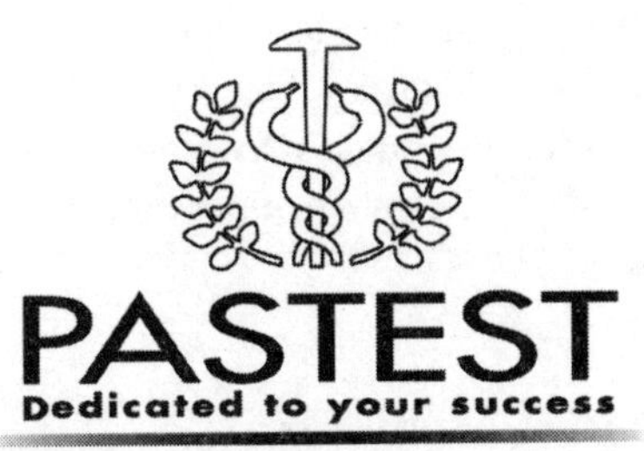

Egerton Court
Parkgate Estate
Knutsford
Cheshire WA16 8DX

Telephone: 01565 752000

First published 2003

ISBN 1 901198 19 7

A catalogue record for this book is available from the British Library.

Typeset by Breeze Limited, Manchester.
Printed by Martins the Printers Limited, Berwick-upon-Tweed

CONTENTS

PREFACE

This book is primarily intended for candidates sitting the System MCQ section of the MRCS/AFRCS examinations. The multiple true false and extended matching questions and practice papers have been specifically structured to reflect the syllabus of all the Surgical Royal Colleges of UK and Ireland.

The goal of such a book is to help assess knowledge and provide an adjunct to reading, in addition to alerting one to areas that require further study. This book covers many of the 'most popular' topics that appear in the MRCS/AFRCS examinations. MCQ practice will increase overall knowledge and detailed explanations have been written to aid revision. The explanations should also be useful to candidates in other parts of the examination.

I hope that this book will not be restricted only to candidates sitting the MRCS/AFRCS examination but will be of use to Final Year medical students.

Christopher L H Chan

CONTRIBUTORS

Contributor Coordinator:

Victoria Chamberlain MB ChB, MRCS, Wellington Hospital, Wellington, New Zealand

Contributors:

Steven J Arnold MSc (Hons), MRCS (Eng), East Surrey Hospital, Redhill, Surrey
Robert Attaran BSc (Hons), MBChB (Hons), University College London Hospital, London
Sunil Auplish MBBS, BSc (Hons), MRCS, Orthopaedic SpR, Oxford rotation
Philip J Blackie BSc (Hons), MBBS (London), Senior House Officer in Anaesthetics, King's College Hopital, London
Victoria Chamberlain MB ChB, MRCS, Wellington Hospital, Wellington, New Zealand
Joseph A Dawson MBBS MRCS (Eng), Basic Surgical Trainee, The Warwickshire & Worcestershire Basic Surgical Training Scheme
Richard J D Hewitt BSc MBBS, Senior House Officer in Neurosurgery, St Bartholomew's and the London Hospitals, London
Kismet Hossain-Ibrahim MBBS, BSc (Hons), MRCS (Eng), MRCS (Ed), Research Assistant, Department of Anatomy, University College London
Stephen J Washington MB ChB, Senior House Officer in Plastic Surgery, Christie Hospital, Manchester

EXAMINATION TECHNIQUE

The MCQ section of the MRCS comprises two written papers, one for the Core modules and another for the System modules. Each paper consists of 65 multiple choice stems and 60 extended matching items. Candidates are allowed 2½ hours per paper.

Pacing yourself accurately during the examination to finish on time, or with time to spare, is essential. There are two common mistakes which cause good candidates to fail the MRCS written examinations. These are neglecting to read the directions and questions carefully enough and failing to fill in the computer answer card properly. You must read the instructions given to candidates at the beginning of each section of the paper to ensure that you complete the answer sheet correctly.

You must also decide on a strategy to follow with regard to marking your answer sheet. The answer sheet is read by an automatic document reader and transfers the information to a computer. It is critical that the answer sheet is filled in clearly and accurately using the pencils provided. Failure to fill in your name and your examination correctly could result in the rejection of your paper.

Some candidates mark their answers directly onto the computer sheet as they go through the question, others prefer to make a note of their answers on the question paper, and reserve time at the end to transfer their answers onto the computer sheet. If you choose the first method, there is a chance that you may decide to change your answer after a second reading. If you do change your answer on the computer sheet, you must ensure that your original is thoroughly erased. If you choose the second method, make sure that you allow enough time to transfer your answers methodically onto the computer sheet, as rushing at this stage could introduce some costly mistakes. You will find it less confusing if you transfer your marks after you have completed each section of the examination. You must ensure that you have left sufficient time to transfer your marks from the question paper to the answer sheet. You should also be aware that no additional time will be given at the end of the examination to allow you to transfer your marks.

If you find that you have time left at the end of the examination, there can be a temptation to re-read your answers time and time again, so that even those that seemed straightforward will start to look less convincing. In this situation, first thoughts are usually best, don't alter your initial answers unless you are sure.

You must also ensure that you read the question (both stem and items) carefully. Regard each item as being independent of every other item, each referring to a specific quantum of knowledge. The item (or the stem and the item taken together) make up a statement as "True" or "False". The number of stems will vary for each question. For this reason, a mark will not necessarily be required for each column of the answer sheet. For every correct answer you will gain a mark (+1). For the MRCS (London) examination, marks will not be deducted for a wrong answer. Equally, you will not gain a mark if you mark both true and false.

The MRCS exams in England are not negatively marked. For this reason you should answer every question as you have nothing to lose. If you do not know the answer to a question, you should make an educated guess – you may well get the answer right and gain a mark.

If you feel that you need to spend more time puzzling over a question, leave it and, if you have time, return to it. Make sure you have collected all the marks you can before you come back to any difficult questions.

Multiple choice questions are not designed to trick you or confuse you, they are designed to test your knowledge of medicine. Accept each question at face value.

The aim of this book is to give you two different methods of revising for the System module paper. Firstly, there are five chapters covering each of the five System modules containing a mixture of MCQs and EMQs. This gives you a range of questions to test your knowledge on specific subjects. These are then followed by two practice papers to give you the chance to experience answering questions in exam format. You could also time yourself to see how well you manage to answer your questions in the 2½ hours allowed.

Working through the questions in this book will help you to identify your weak subject areas. In the last few weeks before the exam it will be important for you to avoid minor unimportant areas and concentrate on the most important subject areas covered in the exam.

ABBREVIATIONS

1,25-DHCC	1,25-dihydroxycholecalciferol
5-FU	5-fluorouracil
A&E	accident and emergency
AAA	abdominal aortic aneurysm
ABC	airway, breathing, circulation
ACL	anterior cruciate ligament
AF	atrial fibrillation
ASIS	anterior superior iliac spine
AST	aspartate aminotransferase (aka serum glutamate oxaloacetate transaminase, SGOT)
AV	arteriovenous
AVF	arteriovenous fistula
AVN	avascular necrosis
AXR	abdominal X-ray
BCG	bacille Calmette-Guérin
BP	blood pressure
CBD	common bile duct
CCF	congestive cardiac failure
CCK	cholecystokinin
CEA	carotid endarterectomy
COPD	chronic obstructive pulmonary disease
CREST	calcinosis, Raynaud's, [o]esophagus scleroderma, telangiectasia [syndrome]
CRP	C-reactive protein
CT	computed tomography
CVA	cardiovascular/cerebrovascular accident
CXR	chest X-ray
DHS	dynamic hip screw
DIC	disseminated intravascular coagulopathy
dl	decilitre; one-tenth of a litre, i.e. 100 ml
DMSA	dimercaptosuccinic acid
DTPA	diethylenetriaminepentaacetic acid
DVT	deep venous thrombosis
ECG	electrocardiogram/aphy
ERCP	endoscopic retrograde cholangiopancreatography
ESR	erythrocyte sedimentation rate
EUA	examination under anaesthesia
FAP	familial adenomatous polyposis
FBC	full blood count
FGF	fibroblast growth factor
FHH	familial hypocalcuric hypercalcaemia

FNAC	fine-needle aspiration cytology
FOB	faecal occult blood
GABA	gamma-aminobutyric acid
GCS	Glasgow Coma Scale
GI	gastrointestinal
GP	general practitioner
GTN	glyceryl trinitrate
h	hour
HIDA	hepatoiminodiacetic acid [lidofenin] [nuclear medicine scan]
HIV	human immunodeficiency virus
HPV	human papillomavirus
IBD	inflammatory bowel disease
IMA	inferior mesenteric artery
ITU	intensive therapy unit
IU	international unit
IV	intravenous
IVC	inferior vena cava
IVU	intravenous urography
kPa	kilopascal
KUB	kidney, ureter, bladder
L	lumbar
LDH	lactate dehydrogenase
LHRH	luteinising hormone-releasing hormone
M_1	degree of metastasis
MAG-3	mercaptoacetyl triglycine
MEN-1	multiple endocrine neoplasia, type 1
MI	myocardial infarction
mmol	millimole
MRA	magnetic resonance angiography
MRI	magnetic resonance imaging
MRSA	methicillin-resistant *Staphylococcus aureus*
MSU	midstream urine
M-VAC	methotrexate–vinblastine, doxorubicin [has replaced Adriamycin®], cisplatin
N_1	degree of nodal involvement
Nd–YAG	neodymium–yttrium aluminium garnet
NEC	necrotising enterocolitis
NICE	National Institute for Clinical Excellence
NO	nitric oxide
NSAID	non-steroidal anti-inflammatory drug
Osm	osmole

PAMAID	Personal Adaptive Mobility Aid for the frail and elderly visually impaired
PAN	polyarteritis nodosa
PCNL	percutaneous nephrolithotomy
$P\text{CO}_2$	partial pressure of carbon dioxide
PDGF	platelet-derived growth factor
PDS	prolonged tensile strength
PE	pulmonary embolism
PMC	pseudomembranous colitis
$P\text{O}_2$	partial pressure of oxygen
PTFE	polytetrafluoroethylene
PTH	parathyroid hormone
PUJ	pelviureteric junction obstruction
RA	rheumatoid arthritis
RIF	right iliac fossa
RTA	road traffic accident
RUQ	right upper quadrant
S	sacral
SGOT	serum glutamate oxaloacetate transaminase (aka aspartate aminotransferase, AST)
SLE	systemic lupus erythematosus
SMA	superior mesenteric artery
SVC	superior vena cava
T1	tumour stage
T3	triiodothyronine
T4	tetraiodothyronine, thyroxine
TB	tuberculosis
TIA	transient ischaemic attack
TPA	tissue plasminogen activator
TPN	total parenteral nutrition
TRH	thyrotropin-releasing hormone
TSH	thyroid-stimulating hormone
TURBT	transurethral resection of a bladder tumour
TURP	transurethral resection of the prostate
U	unit
UC	ulcerative colitis
UDT	undescended testis
UTI	urinary tract infection
VIP	vasoactive intestinal protein
VIPoma	vasoactive intestinal polypeptide-secreting tumour
WBC	white blood cell/count
WCC	white cell count

CHAPTER 1 : LOCOMOTOR

1.1 Theme: Peripheral nerve anatomy

A Saphenous
B Femoral
C Obturator
D Sural
E Common peroneal
F Tibial
G Sciatic
H Medial cutaneous nerve of the thigh
I L5 nerve root
J S1 nerve root

For each of the clinical scenarios below, select the nerve most likely to be involved from the list above. Each option may be used once, more than once, or not at all.

❑ **1.** After removal of a below-knee plaster cast, applied for an Achilles tendon rupture, a 46-year-old man notices that the side of his leg and top of his foot is numb and that he frequently trips while walking, particularly when climbing stairs.

❑ **2.** A 35-year-old woman, who was initially found to have a large left-sided cystic ovarian tumour, now presents with pain radiating down the medial part of her thigh and a 'bearing down' feeling in her pelvis.

❑ **3.** A 25-year-old woman suddenly experiences severe pain in her back with shooting pains passing down the back of her left calf into the lateral part of her left foot. On examination there is loss of the ankle reflex on that side and loss of discriminatory touch over the lateral part and sole of the foot.

❑ **4.** An 18-year-old motorcyclist is involved in an RTA and sustains a fracture dislocation of the right hip. The painful thigh is difficult to examine, but there is an obvious foot drop and sensory loss below the knee except in the skin on the medial part of the leg and foot and upper posterior part of the calf.

1.2 Boundaries of the femoral triangle include the

- ❑ A inguinal ligament
- ❑ B adductor longus
- ❑ C adductor magnus
- ❑ D pectineus
- ❑ E iliopsoas

1.3 The greater sciatic foramen contains the

- ❑ A superior gluteal nerve
- ❑ B sacrotuberous ligament
- ❑ C pudendal nerve
- ❑ D obturator internus tendon
- ❑ E posterior femoral cutaneous nerve

1.4 Theme: Calcium homeostasis

A Primary hyperparathyroidism
B Secondary hyperparathyroidism
C Parathyroid carcinoma
D Hypocalciuric hypercalcaemia
E Multiple myeloma
F Paget's disease

For each of the patients described below, choose the most suitable diagnosis from the list of options above. Each option may be used once, more than once, or not at all.

❑ **1.** A 32-year-old man has a serum Ca^{2+} concentration of 2.8 mmol/l, renal stones and urinary Ca^{2+} level of 2.0 mmol/day with normal PTH levels.

❑ **2.** A 50-year-old man has a corrected serum Ca^{2+} concentration of 2.55 mmol/l, a urinary Ca^{2+} level of 10 mmol/day and an increased PTH level.

❑ **3.** A 40-year-old woman complains of tiredness. She has a corrected serum Ca^{2+} concentration of 2.75 mmol/l and a 24-hour urinary Ca^{2+} collection of 0.5 mmol.

1.5 In the femoral region the

- ❑ A femoral sheath contains the femoral vessels
- ❑ B femoral canal lies lateral to the femoral vein
- ❑ C femoral canal contains Cloquet's lymph node
- ❑ D femoral ring is the abdominal end of the femoral canal
- ❑ E pubic branch of the inferior epigastric vein replaces the obturator vein in 30% of cases

1.6 A positive left Trendelenburg test may be associated with

- ❑ A an injury to the right gluteus medius muscle
- ❑ B a displaced left femoral head
- ❑ C a shortened right femur
- ❑ D an injury to the left abductor muscles
- ❑ E an injury to the left pectineus muscle

1.7 Theme: Shoulder pain

A Supraspinatus tendonitis
B Supraspinatus rupture
C Acute calcific tendonitis
D Biceps rupture
E Acromioclavicular joint dislocation
F Posterior dislocation of the shoulder
G Frozen shoulder

For each of the patients described below, select the most likely diagnosis from the list of options above. Each option may be used once, more than once, or not at all.

❑ **1.** A 52-year-old plasterer presents with a 1-year history of shoulder pain and difficulty in raising his arm. Symptoms have been markedly worse over the last few weeks. On examination he has marked tenderness around the acromium process. He is unable to actively abduct his arm and seems to have developed a special manoeuvre to raise his arm and keep it raised.

❑ **2.** A 32-year-old presents to A&E with a 24-hour history of increasing pain in his shoulder since doing some digging in the garden. He is found to be in excruciating pain and all movements of the shoulder are impossible due to pain. There is a point of exquisite tenderness just inferior to the acromium process.

❑ **3.** An American football player hurt his shoulder during a tackle and presents with deformity over the lateral end of the clavicle. The area is locally tender and swollen.

❑ **4.** A 70-year-old pensioner was advised to start some regular shoulder exercises to help his recovery from a dislocated shoulder. During one lift he felt a snap and developed sudden pain. He has returned to A&E fearing that he has dislocated his shoulder again. Pain and bruising in the upper arm are noted, along with a lump.

❑ **5.** A long-term, poorly controlled epileptic man, presents to his GP with a 1-week history of a stiff painful shoulder. He cannot remember any specific injury. All movements are very restricted and painful.

1.8 Theme: Anatomy of joints in the upper limb

A Shoulder
B Elbow
C Superior radioulnar
D Inferior radioulnar
E Wrist
F Interphalangeal
G First carpometacarpal
H Acromioclavicular

For each of the descriptions below, select the most likely joint from the list above. Each option may be used once, more than once, or not at all.

❑ **1.** Has an intra-articular tendon passing through the joint.

❑ **2.** Is a saddle joint.

❑ **3.** Is stabilised by an annular ligament.

❑ **4.** Movements at this distal joint are the reciprocal of those at the proximal joint.

1.9 Anterior shoulder dislocation

❑ A is less common than posterior shoulder dislocation
❑ B is usually subcoracoid
❑ C usually presents with the arm in the adduction position
❑ D is a recognised cause of axillary nerve palsy
❑ E can be treated using Kocher's manoeuvre

1.10 In compartment syndrome

❑ A there must be an underlying fracture
❑ B loss of a peripheral pulse is an early sign
❑ C the anterior lower leg compartment is rarely affected
❑ D pain on passive dorsiflexion of the toes and the foot suggests that the posterior compartment of the lower leg is involved
❑ E sensory loss occurs distally

1.11 Dupuytren's contracture

❑ A may be associated with an increase in oxygen free radicals
❑ B is not related to alcohol intake
❑ C may be familial
❑ D can occur in the foot
❑ E is treated by limited fasciectomy

1.12 Theme: Bone pathology

A Acute calcific tendonitis
B Osteomyelitis
C Osteosarcoma
D Bone cyst
E Avascular necrosis

For each of the patients described below, select the most likely diagnosis from the list of options above. Each option may be used once, more than once, or not at all.

❑ **1.** A 35-year-old deep-sea diver presents with a 2-week history of right shoulder pain. His X-ray is normal, but MRI shows an increased signal at the head of humerus.

❑ **2.** An 8-year-old boy fractures his humerus in a fall. A plain X-ray shows a radiolucent area with a sclerotic edge at the fracture site.

1.13 Intracapsular femoral neck

- ❑ A has a blood supply from the ligamentum teres
- ❑ B fracture commonly occurs in patients with osteoarthritis
- ❑ C carries an increased risk of non-union
- ❑ D is usually fixed with a dynamic hip screw

1.14 In displaced intracapsular femoral neck fractures

- ❑ A the leg is usually shortened and externally rotated
- ❑ B the injuring force may be trivial
- ❑ C the femoral head is less likely to undergo necrosis than in intertrochanteric fractures
- ❑ D the standard treatment consists of a dynamic hip screw (DHS)
- ❑ E the 6-month mortality rate is less than 10%

1.15 Intertrochanteric fractures of the femur

- ❑ A cause shortening and external rotation of the lower limb
- ❑ B usually cause the leg to become abducted
- ❑ C significantly compromise the blood supply to the femoral head in most cases
- ❑ D are best treated by hemiarthroplasty
- ❑ E are best treated with dynamic hip screw (DHS) fixation

1.16 Carpal tunnel syndrome is associated with

- ❑ A a Colles' fracture
- ❑ B obesity
- ❑ C epilepsy
- ❑ D cervical spondylosis
- ❑ E rheumatoid arthritis

1.17 In supracondylar fractures of the humerus

- ❑ A the patient is typically elderly
- ❑ B the patient has usually fallen onto the outstretched hand with the elbow straight
- ❑ C the distal fragment is usually displaced posteriorly
- ❑ D the median nerve may be damaged
- ❑ E wrist drop is a typical finding

1.18 Theme: Bone tumours

A Osteosarcoma
B Bony metastasis from lung carcinoma
C Myeloma
D Osteochondroma
E Ewing's sarcoma

Select the most appropriate and likely diagnosis from the list above. Each option may be used once, more than once, or not at all.

❑ **1.** A 50-year-old man presents with weakness, lethargy and back pain. X-ray of his back reveals a crush fracture of his vertebra with multiple punched-out defects in his sacrum and ilium. Blood tests reveal an anaemia and a very high ESR. Examination of the urine reveals a Bence-Jones proteinuria.

❑ **2.** A 13-year-old girl presents with a 9-month history of pain in one knee, especially at night. X-ray of her knee shows reactive, new bone formation with periosteal elevation, osteolytic and osteoblastic areas. Only the metaphysis of her tibia is affected.

❑ **3.** A 25-year-old man presents with pain and a visible swelling over his right tibia. X-ray reveals a well-defined bony outgrowth in the metaphysis of his tibia. Clinically the lesion is much larger than the X-ray appearance suggests.

1.19 A flat foot (pes planovalgus) is

❑ A often secondary to peroneus longus damage
❑ B may be associated with tibialis posterior tendon rupture in rheumatoid arthritis
❑ C common in patients with ligamentous laxity
❑ D usually painful
❑ E treated by fusion of the subtalar joint

1.20 The following conditions are commonly associated with significant foot pain:

- ❑ A alcoholic neuropathy
- ❑ B hallux rigidus
- ❑ C L2/L3 disc prolapse
- ❑ D rheumatoid arthritis
- ❑ E Dupuytren's contracture

1.21 Club feet (talipes equinovarus)

- ❑ A are associated with oligohydramnios
- ❑ B have a familial tendency
- ❑ C are most frequent in girls
- ❑ D treatment should be delayed until the child is starting to walk
- ❑ E are associated with spina bifida

1.22 A young lady presents with a history of her left knee giving way as she turns. She recalls twisting her knee during a hockey match. Immediately after, she had severe pain and was unable to weight-bear. The A&E doctor couldn't flex her knee beyond 80° and was unable to extend the knee fully because of pain. An effusion was present. What is/are the most likely possible diagnosis(es)?

- ❑ A Anterior cruciate rupture
- ❑ B Septic arthritis
- ❑ C Medial collateral ligament rupture
- ❑ D Medial meniscal tear
- ❑ E Patella dislocation

1.23 Tourniquet

- ❑ A may be safely inflated for 60 minutes (constant duration) in the upper limb
- ❑ B application does not affect nerve conduction
- ❑ C should be released before a wound is sutured
- ❑ D pressure should be between arterial and venous pressures
- ❑ E is used as part of a Biers' block technique for upper limb anaesthesia

1.24 Risk factors for joint replacement infection include

- ❑ A uncemented prosthesis
- ❑ B psoriasis
- ❑ C diabetes mellitus
- ❑ D *in-situ* urinary catheter
- ❑ E prednisolone

1.25 The following predispose to non-traumatic lateral dislocation of the patella:

- ❑ A prominent lateral femoral condyle
- ❑ B generalised ligamentous laxity
- ❑ C weak vastus lateralis
- ❑ D weak rectus femoris
- ❑ E valgus knee

1.26 Slipped upper femoral epiphysis

- ❑ A is more common in males than females
- ❑ B is a recognised cause of knee pain in the adolescent
- ❑ C is bilateral in 1% of cases
- ❑ D leaves the leg lying short and internally rotated
- ❑ E can lead to avascular necrosis of the femoral head

1.27 In the healing of adult bone

- ❑ A the stimulation of osteoprogenitor cells by factors such as FGF and PDGF play an important role
- ❑ B the histological appearance resembles that in an osteosarcoma
- ❑ C internal fixation reduces callus formation
- ❑ D a fracture haematoma delays healing by maintaining a degree of separation between the bone ends
- ❑ E callus formation can be seen on an X-ray by 10 days

1.28 Late complications of fractures include

- ❑ A infection
- ❑ B Volkmann's ischaemic contracture
- ❑ C tendon rupture
- ❑ D myositis ossificans
- ❑ E algodystrophy

1.29 Fracture non-union

- ❑ A may occur if the fracture surfaces are interposed by muscle
- ❑ B characteristically produces painless movement at the fracture site
- ❑ C always requires treatment
- ❑ D may be treated by electrical stimulation
- ❑ E of the atrophic type may require bone grafting

1.30 Delayed fracture union

- ❑ A is rarely seen in the lower tibia
- ❑ B may be caused by an intact fellow bone
- ❑ C produces a tender fracture site
- ❑ D produces a marked periosteal reaction
- ❑ E may be treated by functional bracing

1.31 Recurrent dislocation of patella

- ❑ A usually occurs towards the lateral side as the knee is flexed
- ❑ B is more common in varus deformity of knee
- ❑ C may give rise to osteoarthritis
- ❑ D has an equal sex incidence
- ❑ E is usually unilateral

1.32 X-ray features of osteoarthritis include

- ❑ A subchondral bone cysts
- ❑ B osteophyte formation
- ❑ C ankylosis
- ❑ D symmetrical joint-space narrowing
- ❑ E periarticular osteoporosis

1.33 Paget's disease of bone

- ❑ A characteristically affects the cortex
- ❑ B can be treated with bisphosphonates
- ❑ C causes an elevated alkaline phosphatase
- ❑ D is uncommon below 50 years of age
- ❑ E is most commonly found in the femur
- ❑ F predisposes to fractures
- ❑ G can be treated with calcium

1.34 In calcium homeostasis

- ❑ A calcitonin reduces renal excretion
- ❑ B calcitonin increases bone resorption
- ❑ C vitamin D is converted to 25-hydroxycholecalciferol in the kidney
- ❑ D vitamin D activation is increased by parathyroid hormone
- ❑ E oestrogen increases calcium absorption

1.35 Tuberculosis of the knee

- ❑ A may begin as a synovitis
- ❑ B rarely causes muscle wasting
- ❑ C causes subarticular bone erosion
- ❑ D produces a marked periosteal reaction
- ❑ E is usually diagnosed by acid-fast bacilli in synovial fluid

1.36 Club foot

- ❑ A is usually held in the equinus position
- ❑ B is usually held in the valgus position
- ❑ C affects girls twice as often as boys
- ❑ D may be associated with neural tube defects
- ❑ E invariably needs surgical correction
- ❑ F is bilateral in one-third of cases

1.37 Postoperative osteomyelitis

- ❑ A often produces tenderness and pain on movement of the limb
- ❑ B may be accurately diagnosed by MRI in the early stages
- ❑ C is more likely if there is implant loosening
- ❑ D is eliminated by prophylactic antibiotics
- ❑ E is usually due to a single bacterial pathogen

1.38 Carpal tunnel syndrome

- ❑ A occurs during pregnancy
- ❑ B is associated with hypothyroidism
- ❑ C characteristically produces pain during the day
- ❑ D produces a positive Froment's sign
- ❑ E may be diagnosed by nerve conduction tests

1.39 Dupuytren's contracture

- ❑ A is inherited as an autosomal recessive trait
- ❑ B has an association with carbamazepine therapy
- ❑ C often causes paraesthesia
- ❑ D should always be corrected
- ❑ E may require digit amputation
- ❑ F is often bilateral

1.40 Humeral shaft fractures

- ❑ A usually require immobilisation in plaster
- ❑ B may cause weakness of the metacarpophalangeal extensors
- ❑ C are associated with delayed union
- ❑ D are uncommon in children <3 years
- ❑ E take approximately 4 weeks to unite

1.41 Perthes' disease

- ❑ A is common in the Afro-Caribbean population
- ❑ B is more common in girls than in boys
- ❑ C affects social class V more than I
- ❑ D has a peak presentation age at 2 years of age
- ❑ E produces limited abduction movement

1.42 Combined fracture of the radius and ulna

- ❑ A in children is usually treated by open reduction and fixation
- ❑ B in adults usually requires open reduction and internal fixation
- ❑ C is commonly associated with posterior interosseus nerve damage
- ❑ D frequently causes ischaemia to the hand
- ❑ E may be complicated by cross-union

1.43 Internal fixation is

- ❑ A often used in the treatment of pathological fractures
- ❑ B useful in the treatment of fractures in the multiply injured patient
- ❑ C occasionally complicated by chronic osteitis
- ❑ D used in the treatment of infected fractures
- ❑ E sometimes complicated by fracture non-union

1.44 The complications of pelvic fractures include

- ❑ A rupture of the internal iliac vein
- ❑ B madura foot
- ❑ C extraperitoneal urinary extravasation
- ❑ D rectal perforation
- ❑ E fat embolus
- ❑ F urethral injury

1.45 In the popliteal fossa the

- ❑ A roof is formed by the fascia lata
- ❑ B sciatic nerve divides into tibial and common peroneal branches at the apex
- ❑ C deepest structure is the popliteal vein
- ❑ D common peroneal nerve is overlain by the semitendinosus muscle
- ❑ E roof is pierced by the saphenous nerve

1.46 In the bony pelvis the

- ❑ A sacral cornua are palpable per rectum
- ❑ B pubic tubercles are palpable lateral to the external ring of the inguinal canal
- ❑ C femoral canals lie medial to the lacunar ligaments
- ❑ D ischial spines are palpable per vaginum
- ❑ E transtubercular plane passes through the spinous process of the L3 vertebra

1.47 The scaphoid bone

- ❑ A articulates with the radius
- ❑ B is palpable in the 'snuffbox'
- ❑ C has a vascular supply penetrating its distal surface
- ❑ D gives attachment to the flexor retinaculum
- ❑ E gives attachment to the adductor pollicis muscle

1.48 On the dorsum of the foot the

- ❑ A dorsalis pedis artery lies medial to the extensor hallucis longus tendon
- ❑ B deep peroneal nerve lies medial to the dorsalis pedis artery
- ❑ C L5 dermatome is present
- ❑ D great saphenous vein lies anterior to the medial malleolus
- ❑ E inferior extensor retinaculum loops under the medial longitudinal arch

1.49 In the lumbosacral plexus the

- ❑ A sympathetic trunk sends grey rami to all roots
- ❑ B parasympathetic nerves originate from S2/3 spinal segments
- ❑ C lumbosacral trunk lies on the piriformis muscle
- ❑ D lumbosacral trunk underlies the common iliac vessels
- ❑ E posterior divisions of anterior rami supply the adductor muscles

1.50 The serratus anterior muscle

- ❑ A has the thoracodorsal nerve deep to its fascia over its lateral surface
- ❑ B rotates the scapula
- ❑ C retracts the scapula
- ❑ D receives its nerve supply from the upper trunk of the brachial plexus
- ❑ E has most of its fibres inserted into the superior angle of the scapula

1.51 The L3 vertebra

- ❑ A undergoes rotatory movements
- ❑ B gives attachment to the left crus of the diaphragm
- ❑ C is supplied by the internal iliac arteries
- ❑ D has a vertebral foramen (central canal) enclosing the sacral segments of the spinal cord
- ❑ E has a lateral process giving attachment to the iliolumbar ligament

1.52 In the antecubital fossa the

- ❑ A median nerve lies lateral to the brachial artery
- ❑ B brachial artery branches into radial and ulnar arteries
- ❑ C posterior interosseous nerve may be found
- ❑ D cephalic vein overlies the bicipital aponeurosis
- ❑ E floor is formed by the brachioradialis muscle

1.53 The carpal tunnel contains the

- ❑ A median nerve
- ❑ B ulnar nerve
- ❑ C flexor digitorum brevis tendon
- ❑ D flexor carpi ulnaris tendon
- ❑ E flexor carpi radialis tendon

1.54 In the femoral triangle the

- ❑ A cribriform fascia transmits the superficial branches of the femoral artery
- ❑ B femoral vein lies adjacent to the femoral nerve
- ❑ C profunda femoris artery lies medial to the femoral artery
- ❑ D femoral sheath extends up to 3 cm beyond the inguinal ligament
- ❑ E deep inguinal nodes lie medial to the femoral vein

1.55 Avascular necrosis is a well-recognised complication of

- ❑ A a fracture of the proximal pole of the scaphoid
- ❑ B a supracondylar fracture of the distal humerus
- ❑ C an intertrochanteric fracture of the femoral neck
- ❑ D a fracture of the talar neck
- ❑ E a fracture of the hook of the hamate

1.56 Compartment syndrome

- ❑ A of the forearm commonly presents with pain on flexion of the fingers
- ❑ B commonly occurs with a grade 3b open fracture of the tibia and fibula
- ❑ C is associated with an early reduction in the volume of the distal pulses
- ❑ D may occur following a soft tissue injury without a fracture
- ❑ E is diagnosed by an intracompartmental pressure reading within 30 mmHg of the systolic blood pressure

1.57 The patellar reflex is

- ❑ A lost after femoral nerve transection
- ❑ B mediated through the posterior divisions of anterior rami of lumbar nerves
- ❑ C lost following T12 cord transection
- ❑ D present after L2–4 dorsal root avulsions
- ❑ E absent after dorsal column demyelination

1.58 Common early signs of suppurative tenosynovitis of the flexor tendons of the hand include

- ❑ A the affected finger held in full flexion
- ❑ B a swinging pyrexia
- ❑ C pain on passive finger movement
- ❑ D fusiform swelling of the finger
- ❑ E tenderness of the palm

1.59 Theme: Knee injuries

A Medial meniscus tear
B Medial collateral ligament injury
C Lateral collateral ligament injury
D Patella fracture
E Anterior cruciate ligament tear
F Posterior cruciate ligament tear

For each of the patients described below, select the most likely diagnosis from the list of options above. Each option may be used once, more than once, or not at all.

❑ **1.** A young footballer injured his right knee during a tackle. He managed to continue playing, but over the next few days his knee became increasingly swollen and gave way occasionally. When he presented to A&E, a boggy swelling of the knee was noted. The area of maximal tenderness was about 2 cm above the medial joint line, and valgus strain to the knee demonstrated laxity with the joint 'opened up' and looked deformed.

❑ **2.** A 60-year-old man caught his foot on an uneven paving stone and fell to the ground hitting his knee in the process. His knee became bruised and swollen. He subsequently had difficulty walking. In A&E, it was noted that he had difficulty lifting his leg on and off the couch.

❑ **3.** A driver involved in a head-on collision hit his knee on the dashboard. He sustained a fracture dislocation of the hip and a developed a swollen, painful knee. Several months later he continued to have discomfort in the knee; on review he commented that he still had difficulty going down stairs as he felt 'unsafe' on his knee.

❑ **4.** A young rugby player injured his left knee in a tackle. He completed the game but was aware that his knee was swelling rapidly. He went straight to A&E where a haemarthrosis was drained. No laxity was demonstrated, but 3 months later he is complaining of episodes of giving way, recurrent swelling and discomfort.

❑ **5.** A 13-year-old girl fell whilst practising a dance step on the ice. She immediately became aware of pain on the medial aspect of her knee and had difficulty straightening this knee for a few days. Some weeks later she saw her GP. She was unable to extend her knee fully, and it remained tender on the medial side and with episodes of clicking and pain.

1.60 Theme: Shoulder pain

A Acute calcific tendonitis
B Osteomyelitis
C Osteosarcoma
D Bone cyst
E Avascular necrosis
F Osteochondroma

For each of the patients described below, select the most likely diagnosis from the list of options above. Each option may be used once, more than once, or not at all.

❑ **1.** A 35-year-old oil company executive presents with a 2-week history of right shoulder pain. He has had a renal transplant in the past and has a long history of immunosuppressive medication. On examination there was some restriction of movement. The X-rays were reported as being normal, but an MRI showed abnormalities of the humeral head.

❑ **2.** An 8-year-old boy fell off his bunk bed and sustained a fracture of his proximal humerus. The X-ray confirmed a fracture through a radiolucent lesion with a well-defined sclerotic margin.

❑ **3.** A 14-year-old girl had complained of pain in her shoulder over the preceding 2 weeks before she heard a crack and developed acute pain after lifting her sports bag out of the car. An X-ray confirmed a fracture through an ill-defined lytic lesion of the proximal humerus.

❑ **4.** A 3-year-old boy presented to casualty with a 2-day history of pain in the arm, probably following a tumble down the stairs. He had been miserable for the last 10 days with a temperature, cough and cold. All movements of the shoulder were restricted and associated with pain. His X-ray showed no obvious fracture, but a bony abnormality of the proximal humerus was noted.

1.61 Fracture of the lower end of the ulna

- ❑ A classically occurs after falling on the outstretched hand
- ❑ B impairs pronation
- ❑ C impairs adduction of the wrist
- ❑ D impairs movements of the little finger
- ❑ E involves the wrist joint

1.62 The biceps tendon reflex tests the integrity of the

- ❑ A musculocutaneous nerve
- ❑ B medial cord of the brachial plexus
- ❑ C C5 spinal segment
- ❑ D C6 dorsal root
- ❑ E middle trunk of the brachial plexus

1.63 Theme: Femoral fractures

A Denham pin
B Sliding compression screw with 2-hole plate
C Cannulated screw fixation
D Total hip replacement
E Austin–Moore hemiarthroplasty
F Intramedullary femoral nail
G Reconstruction femoral nail

For each of the clinical situations below, select the most appropriate operation from the above list. Each option may be used once, more than once, or not at all.

❑ **1.** A 75-year-old man fell down the stairs on to his left side. He is admitted to the A&E department complaining of left hip pain. X-rays of the left hip reveal a Garden IV femoral neck fracture.

❑ **2.** A 32-year-old man involved in an RTA is noted to have a Garden II fracture of his right hip with minimal displacement.

❑ **3.** A 65-year-old woman slipped on the pavement and fell on to her right side. X-rays of her right hip reveal an intertrochanteric fracture.

❑ **4.** A 59-year-old cyclist involved in an RTA sustained a left subcapital femoral fracture with minimal displacement and a middle third femoral shaft fracture.

1.64 The fingers are extended after

❑ A contraction of the lumbrical muscles
❑ B contraction of the interosseous muscles
❑ C motor stimulation through the posterior cord of the brachial plexus
❑ D motor stimulation through palmar digital branches of the median nerve
❑ E motor stimulation through the ulnar nerve

1.65 The following conditions are recognised causes of avascular necrosis in the absence of injury:

❑ A sickle-cell disease
❑ B haemophilia A
❑ C Hunter's disease
❑ D Gaucher's disease
❑ E decompression sickness

1.66 Theme: Nerve injury in the arm

A Median nerve injury at the level of the flexor retinaculum
B Radial nerve injury in the radial groove
C Ulnar nerve injury at the wrist
D Ulnar nerve injury at the elbow
E Radial nerve injury at the elbow
F Posterior interosseous nerve and superficial radial nerve injury in the forearm

From the description of the motor and sensory losses below, pick the most appropriate option. Each option may be used once, more than once, or not at all.

❑ **1.** Following a stab wound, a patient has loss of extension of the metacarpophalangeal joints. There is loss of sensation to the skin over both the radial side of the dorsum of the hand, and the anatomical snuffbox. However, wrist extension is preserved.

❑ **2.** A patient presents with an inability to adduct and abduct the fingers, positive Froment's sign, loss of sensation of the medial 1.5 digits and clawing of the ring and little fingers.

1.67 A deep laceration into the thenar eminence could damage the

- ❑ A superficial palmar arterial arch
- ❑ B muscular recurrent branch of the median nerve
- ❑ C radial artery
- ❑ D flexor digitorum superficialis tendons
- ❑ E adductor pollicis muscle

1.68 During full abduction of the arm the following muscles are active:

- ❑ A infraspinatus
- ❑ B trapezius
- ❑ C supraspinatus
- ❑ D serratus anterior
- ❑ E teres major

1.69 In a patient with a prolapsed L5/S1 intervertebral disc

- ❑ A there may be no history of trauma
- ❑ B pain radiating to the buttocks implies nerve root involvement
- ❑ C pain radiating down to the ankle on coughing and sneezing implies nerve root involvement
- ❑ D urinary retention can be secondary to pain and bedrest
- ❑ E an absent ankle jerk means that the disc should be removed

1.70 The radiological features of osteoarthritis include

- ❑ A an increase in the joint space due to synovial fluid production
- ❑ B bony sclerosis
- ❑ C cyst formation in the weight-bearing portion of the joint
- ❑ D osteophyte formation at the joint margin
- ❑ E erosions in the periarticular region

1.71 Fat embolism

- ❑ A is associated with diabetes
- ❑ B only follows lower limb fractures
- ❑ C may produces fat in the urine
- ❑ D does not occur in compound fractures
- ❑ E produces petechial brain haemorrhages

1.72 Management of a compound fracture of the proximal femur includes

- ❑ A application of a plaster cast
- ❑ B antitetanus toxoid
- ❑ C oral antibiotics
- ❑ D iodine dressing to wound
- ❑ E assessment of the Glasgow Coma Scale (GCS)

1.73 Theme: Back pain

A Prolapsed intervertebral disc
B Scheuermann's disease
C TB of the spine
D Spondylolysis
E Discitis
F Facet joint arthritis
G Idiopathic scoliosis

For each of the patients described below, select the most likely diagnosis from the list of options above. Each option may be used once, more than once, or not at all.

❑ **1.** An 18-year-old student who is a fast bowler for his college cricket team has had increasing back pain for the last few weeks of the season. Attempts at bowling have been associated with severe acute pain. He is noted to have a slight lumbar scoliosis and a stiff lumbar spine. There are no nerve root signs.

❑ **2.** A 20-year-old patient's back pain returned 2 days after a microdiscectomy for a prolapsed intervertebral disc. Over the next 24 hours the pain got progressively worse and he started to feel unwell. His back was stiff and the straight leg raise was limited, but there were no abnormal neurological signs. CRP 100 μg/l, ESR 54 mm/h, WBC 10.5×10^9/l.

❑ **3.** A 16-year-old boy is keen on computers and avoids all physical activities. He has had pain in the upper part of his back for some months and has been told it is due to 'growing pains'. His parents are worried about his posture. The GP has noted a curvature of the spine and arranged an X-ray, whereupon the diagnosis became obvious.

❑ **4.** A 16-year-old boy immigrated to the UK 3 years ago from India. He has been troubled with back pain for several years, but since working in his father's shop it has deteriorated. He now feels constantly tired and has been losing weight.

❑ **5.** A 60-year-old man spent all day helping his son lay a patio garden. The following morning he was in severe pain from his back. The pain radiated to the buttocks and into his thighs. He was barely able to get out of bed. His GP was called but by the time he had arrived the pain had eased slightly.

1.74 Common indications for considering internal fixation of fractures include

❑ A pathological fractures
❑ B intra-articular fractures
❑ C open fractures
❑ D post open exploration of a concomitant vascular injury
❑ E failure to achieve a closed reduction of a simple closed fracture

1.75 The following structures exit the greater sciatic foramen below the piriformis muscle:

❑ A superior gluteal nerve and artery
❑ B nerve to obturator internus
❑ C femoral cutaneous nerve
❑ D inferior gluteal nerve
❑ E posterior cutaneous nerve of the thigh

1.76 The tibial nerve in the popliteal fossa

❑ A runs superficial to the popliteal vessels
❑ B emerges medial to the popliteal artery
❑ C gives off the sural nerve as a branch
❑ D supplies muscles for dorsiflexion of ankle
❑ E supplies the popliteus
❑ F runs deep to the gastrocnemius

1.77 Theme: Bone disease

A Paget's disease
B Avascular necrosis
C Rickets
D Osteomalacia
E Osteoarthritis
F Osteosarcoma
G Osteochondroma

For each of the clinical scenarios given below, select the most likely diagnosis from the list above. Each option may be used once, more than once, or not at all.

❑ **1.** A patient with a successful renal transplant presented with severe hip pain. She had been treated with immunosuppressive drugs and steroids for many years prior to her transplant 10 years ago.

❑ **2.** A 15-year-old boy was kicked when playing football, and ever since he has been aware that his lower thigh has been painful and swollen. Examination confirmed a diffuse swelling and tenderness around the distal femur with a small effusion of the knee with noticeable muscle wasting.

❑ **3.** A 2-year-old toddler was referred for advice regarding bow-legs. These were considered to be within normal limits for his age, but he was also noted to be of short stature and had a past medical history which included a period of 'failure to thrive'. This, however, appeared to improve on monitoring without the need for formal investigation.

❑ **4.** A 60-year-old man came to clinic asking for advice regarding his 'bent' legs. The history was difficult to elicit because of his deafness. But it appeared that his legs had become progressively deformed over the last few years, although with little in the way of pain.

❑ **5.** A 22-year-old man wanted advice regarding a lump in his axilla which was bony, hard and non-tender. It had been present for many years and with no changes in characteristics recently. Thorough examination confirmed the presence of several bony swellings in the metaphyseal region of several bones.

1.78 Acute osteomyelitis

- ❑ A is usually caused by *Streptococcus pyogenes*
- ❑ B may occur from a skin abrasion
- ❑ C usually begins in the metaphysis
- ❑ D is more common in the vertebrae in adults
- ❑ E has normal X-ray appearances during the first 10 days

CHAPTER 2: VASCULAR

2.1 The IVC

- ❑ A enters the thoracic cavity at the level of T8
- ❑ B commences at the level of L5
- ❑ C receives bilateral gonadal venous drainage directly
- ❑ D lies anterior to the aorta
- ❑ E lies to the right of the aorta
- ❑ F lies posterior to the caudate lobe of the liver

2.2 The middle meningeal artery

- ❑ A arises from the maxillary branch of the external carotid artery
- ❑ B originates in the pterygopalatine fossa
- ❑ C enters the skull through the foramen ovale
- ❑ D supplies the dura mater
- ❑ E rupture of this artery is associated with an extradural haematoma

2.3 Theme: Anatomy of the pelvic vasculature

A Superior gluteal artery
B Superior vesical artery
C Gonadal veins
D Superior rectal vein
E Inferior vesical artery
F Lateral sacral veins
G Internal iliac artery
H Uterine artery

For each of the statements below, select the most likely option from the list above. Each option may be used once, more than once, or not at all.

❑ **1.** Communicates with the vertebral venous plexus.

❑ **2.** Forms the medial umbilical ligament.

❑ **3.** Supplies the prostate gland.

❑ **4.** Drains into the hepatic portal system.

2.4 Direct branches of the coeliac plexus include the

- ❑ A splenic artery
- ❑ B hepatic artery
- ❑ C superior pancreaticoduodenal artery
- ❑ D right gastric artery
- ❑ E gastroduodenal artery

2.5 The right common carotid artery

- ❑ A bifurcates at the level of the upper border of the cricoid cartilage
- ❑ B is a branch of the aortic arch
- ❑ C has the cervical sympathetic chain as an anterior relation
- ❑ D lies lateral to the lateral lobe of the thyroid gland
- ❑ E is separated from the phrenic nerve by the prevertebral fascia
- ❑ F is enclosed within the carotid sheath throughout

2.6 The basilic vein

- ❑ A begins on the medial side of the dorsal venous arch
- ❑ B drains into the subclavian vein
- ❑ C is accompanied by the medial cutaneous nerve of the forearm
- ❑ D pierces the deep fascia in the arm
- ❑ E lies medial to the biceps tendon in the cubital fossa

2.7 The posterior tibial artery

- ❑ A descends on the posterior surface of the tibia distally
- ❑ B gives rise to the anterior tibial artery
- ❑ C gives rise to the peroneal artery
- ❑ D passes anterior to the fibrous arch of the soleus muscle
- ❑ E passes deep to the flexor retinaculum at the ankle

2.8 Theme: Aortic bypass grafting

A Aortobifemoral bypass
B Axillobifemoral bypass
C Left iliac angioplasty
D Left iliac angioplasty and femoral crossover
E Femoral-to-femoral crossover

For each of the patients described below, select the procedure of choice from the list of options above. Each option may be used once, more than once, or not at all.

❑ **1.** A 50-year-old man has a 50-yard (~45 m) claudication distance, with complete occlusion of the lower aorta, with patent femoral vessels.

❑ **2.** A 79-year-old man with emphysema requires home oxygen. He has complete occlusion of the aorta, with patent femoral vessels. His toes appear gangrenous and dusky.

❑ **3.** A 43-year-old postman, otherwise fit and well, who is a non-smoker presents with acute onset claudication in both feet – he is determined to go back to work. He has an aortic bifurcation block with good femoral run-off on both sides.

2.9 Theme: Lower limb ischaemia

A Femoropopliteal bypass
B Percutaneous balloon angioplasty
C Femorodistal bypass
D Below-knee amputation
E Tissue plasminogen activator (TPA) infusion (intra-arterial)
F Fasciotomy
G Lifestyle changes only

For each of the presentations below, select the most likely single treatment from the options listed above. Each option may be used once, more than once, or not at all.

❑ **1.** A 65-year-old man presents with intermittent claudication of the left calf. His claudication distance is 50 yards (~45 m). Angiography demonstrates a 1.5-cm stenosis of the left superficial femoral artery.

❑ **2.** A 73-year-old diabetic woman presents with critical ischaemia of the right lower leg. Angiography reveals extensive disease of the superficial femoral, popliteal and tibial arteries. Pulse-generated, run-off assessment indicates a good run-off in the posterior tibial artery.

❑ **3.** A 72-year-old man presents with a 4-hour history of acute ischaemia of the left leg. Clinical examination demonstrates signs of acute ischaemia with no evidence of gangrene, mottling or neurological deficit. An urgent angiogram reveals a complete thrombotic occlusion of the distal superficial femoral artery.

❑ **4.** A 57-year-old smoker has a history of intermittent claudication of his right calf. His claudication distance is 0.5 mile (~0.8 km). Angiography reveals a 12-cm stenosis in the proximal superficial femoral artery. This has had no effect on his lifestyle, work or social activities.

❑ **5.** A 21-year-old motorcyclist presents with multiple injuries following a road traffic accident. Clinical examination reveals a critically ischaemic right lower leg. The right dorsalis pedis pulse is weak. His right calf is tense and swollen. The intracompartmental pressure is 55 mmHg. Angiography shows no discontinuity of the arterial tree.

2.10 The abdominal aorta

- ❑ A enters the abdomen at the level of the T12 vertebra
- ❑ B divides at the level of the L5 vertebra
- ❑ C lies to the left of the cisterna chyli
- ❑ D gives off 4 single ventral gut arteries
- ❑ E lies posterior to the right renal vein
- ❑ F pulsations are normally palpable

2.11 The femoral artery

- ❑ A underlies the inguinal ligament medial to the deep inguinal ring
- ❑ B supplies the hamstring muscles
- ❑ C supplies the head of the femur
- ❑ D passes through the adductor longus muscle
- ❑ E is subcutaneous in the femoral triangle

2.12 Theme: Lower limb venous disease

A Elevation, rest, NSAIDs and antibiotics
B Emergency surgery
C IV heparin
D Compression bandaging
E Warfarinisation

For each of the patients described below, select the treatment of choice from the list of options above. Each option may be used once, more than once, or not at all.

❑ **1.** A woman has thrombosed varicose veins and cellulitis.

❑ **2.** A woman 5 days after surgery develops a swollen and tender left leg.

❑ **3.** A 64-year-old woman with a known case of venous insufficiency presents with hypotension and profuse bleeding from the medial malleolus of right leg. Conservative treatment has failed.

2.13 The portal vein

- ❑ A is formed behind the body of the pancreas
- ❑ B lies anteriorly to the free edge of the lesser omentum
- ❑ C drains the spleen
- ❑ D forms the central vein of each liver lobule
- ❑ E lies to the right of the superior mesenteric artery
- ❑ F is about 10 cm in length

2.14 Theme: Carotid artery disease

A CT scan
B Carotid Doppler
C ECG
D Carotid angiogram

What initial investigation would you perform for each of the patients listed below? Each option may be used once, more than once, or not at all.

- ❑ **1.** A 71-year-old man presents with a normal pulse, left carotid bruit and left TIAs.

- ❑ **2.** A 71-year-old man presents with a normal pulse, left carotid bruit and a dense left hemiplegia.

2.15 Application of arterial clips during total thyroidectomy could injure the following nerves:

- ❑ A recurrent laryngeal
- ❑ B internal laryngeal
- ❑ C external laryngeal
- ❑ D phrenic
- ❑ E transverse cervical

2.16 The brachial artery is

- ❑ A palpable in the arm
- ❑ B crossed anteriorly by the median nerve
- ❑ C overlain by the biceps tendon
- ❑ D surrounded by venae comitantes
- ❑ E accompanied by the ulnar nerve

2.17 Theme: Investigation of carotid artery disease

A Duplex Doppler ultrasound of carotid arteries
B Carotid angiography
C CT scan of head
D Magnetic resonance angiography (MRA)
E Transcranial Doppler ultrasound
F Near-infrared spectroscopy

From each of the statements below, select the most appropriate investigation from the list above. Each option may be used once, more than once, or not at all.

❑ **1.** What should be the first-line (initial) investigation in a 65-year-old man presenting with an episode of amaurosis fugax affecting his right eye?

❑ **2.** Which is the most appropriate for a 28-year-old woman who collapses with a possible dense, right-sided stroke?

❑ **3.** Which is the most appropriate for intraoperative monitoring during carotid endarterectomy?

2.18 The breast

❑ A has an arterial supply derived from the axillary artery
❑ B is drained by the internal thoracic vein
❑ C has a nipple in the T3 dermatome
❑ D drains 75% of its lymph via the axillary lymph nodes
❑ E has a retromammary space over the pectoralis minor muscle

2.19 The thoracic duct

❑ A runs to the right of the descending aorta
❑ B opens into the superior vena cava
❑ C is anterior to the subclavian artery
❑ D starts at the level of T10
❑ E drains into the right subclavian vein

2.20 Lymphoedema

- ❑ A is usually painful
- ❑ B may follow a venous thrombosis
- ❑ C may be confirmed by duplex ultrasound
- ❑ D rarely responds to active conservative treatment
- ❑ E responds well to diuretic treatment

2.21 Lymphoedema of a single limb

- ❑ A responds well to pneumatic compressions
- ❑ B improves with superficial vein ligation
- ❑ C is associated with lymphatic hypoplasia
- ❑ D renders patients more susceptible to streptococcal infections
- ❑ E can be treated by excising the lymph-drain system

2.22 Lymphatic ducts

- ❑ A contract due to filling
- ❑ B have no valves
- ❑ C lymphoedema occurs secondary to obstruction
- ❑ D have a parasympathetic innervation
- ❑ E empty by pump action of the calf muscles
- ❑ F dilate in oedema

2.23 Recurrent varicose veins

- ❑ A are more common if the long saphenous vein is not tied flush in the first procedure
- ❑ B are more common if incompetent perforators are not identified at the first procedure
- ❑ C should be investigated with duplex Doppler ultrasound
- ❑ D can be treated with sclerotherapy

2.24 Surgery for varicose veins affecting the long saphenous system

- ❑ A the skin incision is placed lateral to the femoral artery
- ❑ B a vertical incision is used routinely
- ❑ C the saphenofemoral junction is usually 3–4 cm inferolateral to the pubic tubercle
- ❑ D there are usually 4 named tributaries
- ❑ E the long saphenous vein must be stripped from ankle to groin to avoid damage to the saphenous nerve

2.25 Abdominal aortic aneurysm

- ❑ A typically rupture at 4-cm diameter
- ❑ B extends above the renal artery in 20% of cases
- ❑ C is invariably visible on abdominal X-ray
- ❑ D is associated with coronary artery disease
- ❑ E has an association with smoking

2.26 Theme: Lymph nodes

A Para-aortic
B Superficial inguinal
C Deep inguinal
D External iliac
E Supraclavicular

For each of the conditions listed below, choose the area in which lymphadenopathy would be most likely to occur. Each option may be used once, more than once, or not at all.

- ❑ **1.** A 20-year-old man with testicular teratoma.
- ❑ **2.** A 40-year-old woman with cervical cancer.
- ❑ **3.** A young man with a perianal abscess.
- ❑ **4.** An 80-year-old man with rectal carcinoma.

2.27 The abdominal aorta

- ❑ A passes into the abdomen at the level of T12
- ❑ B lies to the left of the cysterna chyli
- ❑ C is anterior to the right lumbar sympathetic trunk
- ❑ D gives off 4 paired branches
- ❑ E bifurcates at the level of L5

2.28 Consent for carotid endarterectomy should include

- ❑ A possibility of perioperative stroke
- ❑ B possibility of future stroke
- ❑ C long-term use of antiplatelet aggregation drugs
- ❑ D risk of facial nerve palsy

2.29 Structures encountered on right carotid endarterectomy include

❑ A vagus nerve
❑ B sympathetic chain
❑ C cervical ganglion
❑ D thoracic duct
❑ E pleural membranes

2.30 Theme: Types of ulceration

A Curling's ulcer
B Cushing's ulcer
C Marjolin's ulcer
D Neuropathic ulcers
E Pyoderma gangrenosum

For each of the clinical scenarios listed below, select the lesion most likely to occur in that scenario from the list above. Each option may be used once, more than once, or not at all.

❑ **1.** Squamous-cell carcinoma in a chronic venous ulcer.

❑ **2.** Head injury.

❑ **3.** Major burns.

❑ **4.** Inflammatory bowel disease.

2.31 Saphenofemoral incompetence

❑ A can be assessed by the Brodie–Trendelenburg test
❑ B can be treated with saphenopopliteal ligation
❑ C can be treated by sclerotherapy
❑ D can be treated by the Trendelenburg procedure
❑ E a cough impulse may be transmitted to the long saphenous varicosities

2.32 The cephalic vein

- ❑ A forms in the anatomical snuffbox
- ❑ B is deep to the cutaneous nerve of the forearm
- ❑ C joins the brachial artery at the elbow
- ❑ D is medial to the biceps tendon
- ❑ E forms the axillary vein by joining the basilic vein
- ❑ F has no valves

2.33 When performing a below-knee amputation for ischaemia

- ❑ A the postoperative mortality is approximately 10%
- ❑ B the tibia should be divided about 15 cm below the knee joint
- ❑ C the anterior border of the tibia should be bevelled
- ❑ D nerves should be cut cleanly under tension
- ❑ E a local anaesthetic infusion into the tibial nerve aids postoperative pain relief

2.34 Lower limb arterial bypass grafts

- ❑ A the best patency rates are achieved using autologous saphenous vein
- ❑ B in-situ saphenous vein achieves better patency rates than reversed saphenous vein
- ❑ C cephalic vein is an unsuitable conduit for use in the leg
- ❑ D polytetrafluoroethylene (PTFE) grafts become fully endothelialised in due course
- ❑ E the use of processed human umbilical vein is limited by its inherent antigenicity

2.35 Arch of the aorta

- ❑ A lies wholly in the superior mediastinum
- ❑ B reaches the vertebral column at the lower border of the 4th thoracic vertebra
- ❑ C is crossed anteriorly by the left phrenic nerve
- ❑ D gives rise to the right internal mammary artery
- ❑ E gives rise to the left vertebral artery

2.36 In acute ischaemia of the lower limb

❑ A nerve function is normally maintained for up to 3 hours
❑ B striated muscle recovers well with minimal scarring
❑ C the hallucis longus muscle is the last to recover
❑ D compartment syndrome is rare in established cases
❑ E reperfusion of an ischaemic limb may be a cause of cardiac arrest

2.37 Theme: Vascular tumours

A Kaposi's sarcoma
B Angiosarcoma
C Chemodectoma
D Glomus jugulare tumour
E Leiomyomas

Match the most appropriate feature above with the list below. Each option may be used once, more than once, or not at all.

❑ **1.** Carotid artery.

❑ **2.** Rapid growing, bulky.

❑ **3.** Blue/red macule with HIV.

❑ **4.** Buzzing sensation in head.

2.38 Venous ulceration

❑ A may be associated with Klippel–Trenaunay syndrome
❑ B should be managed by stripping the superficial varicosities in all cases
❑ C is more common in men
❑ D should be investigated by examination of the deep system in all cases
❑ E should not be biopsied as the cause is usually obvious

2.39 In primary lymphoedema of the legs

❑ A there is atrophy of the epidermal lymphatic systems
❑ B malignant infiltration of inguinal lymph nodes is the most common cause
❑ C skin ulcers are uncommon
❑ D treatment with diuretics is of little use
❑ E lymph vesicles and fistulas usually require operative treatment

2.40 Theme: Leg ulcers

A Arterial
B Venous
C Diabetic
D Postphlebitic
E Neoplastic

For each of the patient scenarios below, select the aetiology of the most likely ulcer from the list above. Each option may be used once, more than once, or not at all.

❑ **1.** A 72-year-old woman presents with a 2-year history of an intermittently healing, shallow ulcer above the right medial malleolus. The surrounding skin has a brown discoloration. Ten years previously, she was involved in an RTA and sustained pelvic fractures, which were treated with traction and bedrest.

❑ **2.** A 68-year-old man presents with a deep, painless ulcer beneath the heel of his right foot, which has gradually deteriorated in the 2 months since his admission for pneumonia. The ulcer is surrounded by wet macerated skin and culture has grown MRSA and *Pseudomonas* spp.

❑ **3.** A 94-year-old man presents with a deep, painful ulcer at the tip of his great toe. He has gradually been getting less mobile over the last few months and the pain in his toe stops him from sleeping.

2.41 Carotid artery stenosis

- ❑ A of greater than 50% produces a 10% risk/year of stroke
- ❑ B is closely associated with coronary atherosclerosis
- ❑ C may be reliably diagnosed by auscultation alone
- ❑ D of >90% is most easily diagnosed by duplex ultrasound
- ❑ E of 30–69% and symptomatic should undergo endarterectomy

2.42 Arteriovenous (AV) fistulas

- ❑ A may give a positive Branham's test
- ❑ B may ulcerate, causing haemorrhage
- ❑ C usually improve in pregnancy
- ❑ D may cause multiple embolic events
- ❑ E are a feature of Klippel–Trenaunay syndrome

2.43 Complications following carotid endarterectomy are more common in patients who

- ❑ A are male
- ❑ B are >75 years
- ❑ C have ipsilateral external carotid stenosis
- ❑ D have a history of ischaemic stroke
- ❑ E have systolic hypertension

2.44 Raynaud's phenomenon may be associated with the following:

- ❑ A dysphagia
- ❑ B occupation
- ❑ C warm agglutinins
- ❑ D cutaneous discoloration
- ❑ E Buerger's disease

2.45 Glomus tumours

- ❑ A are usually painless
- ❑ B are more common in men
- ❑ C are blue in colour
- ❑ D may cause phalyngeal changes on X-ray
- ❑ E are treated with radiotherapy

2.46 Venous ulceration

- ❑ A typically occurs on the lateral side of the lower limb above the ankle
- ❑ B may be secondary to deep venous thrombosis
- ❑ C predisposes to malignant change
- ❑ D is more common in men
- ❑ E may be precipitated by minor trauma

2.47 Iodine (^{125}I) fibrinogen uptake test for DVT

- ❑ A may take up to 48 hours to perform
- ❑ B has less sensitivity in the calf than Doppler ultrasound
- ❑ C is most useful as a research tool
- ❑ D may lead to a false-positive result in patients with rheumatoid arthritis
- ❑ E is sometimes used following total hip replacement

2.48 Chemodectomas

- ❑ A arise from preganglionic chromaffin cells
- ❑ B commonly occur in populations living at high altitude
- ❑ C are non-secretory
- ❑ D may be bilateral
- ❑ E commonly metastasise
- ❑ F should be assessed preoperatively by angiography
- ❑ G may be associated with phaeochromocytomas

2.49 The following are recognised causes of leg ulceration in the gaiter region:

- ❑ A tuberculosis
- ❑ B chronic venous insufficiency
- ❑ C short saphenous vein incompetence
- ❑ D ergot poisoning
- ❑ E rheumatoid arthritis

2.50 The following are causes of leg lymphoedema:

- ❑ A familial predisposition
- ❑ B angio-oedema
- ❑ C *Wuchereria bancrofti* infection
- ❑ D radiotherapy
- ❑ E Klippel–Trenaunay syndrome

2.51 In vascular thrombosis

- ❑ A 'coralline clot' is also known as 'red thrombus'
- ❑ B 'propagative clot' is also known as 'white thrombus'
- ❑ C 'red thrombus' has little adherence to the vessel wall and is particularly likely to break up and form emboli
- ❑ D anticoagulants have little effect on platelet aggregation
- ❑ E thrombophlebitis is associated with a clinical inflammatory reaction

2.52 Complications of carotid endarterectomy include

- ❑ A ipsilateral hypoglossal nerve injury
- ❑ B ipsilateral glossopharyngeal nerve injury
- ❑ C ipsilateral facial nerve injury
- ❑ D stridor
- ❑ E postoperative hypertension

2.53 Critical leg ischaemia

- ❑ A is defined as persistently recurring rest pain requiring adequate analgesia for more than 2 months with an ankle systolic pressure of <50 mmHg and/or a toe systolic pressure of <30 mmHg
- ❑ B is defined as ulceration or gangrene of foot or toes with an ankle systolic pressure of <50 mmHg and/or a toe pressure of <30 mmHg
- ❑ C is defined as persistently recurring rest pain requiring adequate analgesia for more than 1 week, with associated ulceration or gangrene of the foot and toes, with an ankle systolic pressure of <70 mmHg and/or a toe pressure of <40 mmHg
- ❑ D can be treated by intra-arterial thrombolysis
- ❑ E with digital gangrene can be effectively treated with lumbar sympathectomy

2.54 Theme: Site of arterial disease

A Lower aorta
B External iliac arteries
C Common femoral arteries
D Profunda femoral arteries
E Left superficial femoral artery
F Right internal iliac artery
G Right peroneal artery
H Right superficial femoral artery

For each of the clinical presentations below, select the most likely site of arterial disease from the list above. Each option may be used once, more than once, or not at all.

❑ **1.** A heavy smoker presented with a history of buttock claudication and impotence.

❑ **2.** An elderly diabetic woman presented with gangrene of her right hallux.

2.55 Regarding vascular lesions of the skin

❑ A naevus flammeus (salmon patch) is the common birthmark
❑ B port-wine stains show little tendency to regress with time
❑ C spider naevi are venular in origin
❑ D juvenile haemangiomas usually involute by the age of 7 years
❑ E cavernous haemangiomas usually involute with time

2.56 Congenital lymphoedema

❑ A may be treated by the Charles' operation
❑ B is due to disease of superficial lymphatics
❑ C may present after 30 years of age
❑ D is more common in women
❑ E is relieved by lymphovenous anastomosis

2.57 The radial artery

- ❑ A anastomoses with the ulnar artery
- ❑ B passes over the trapezium in the wrist
- ❑ C passes into the hand between the two heads of the adductor pollicis muscle
- ❑ D lies lateral to the biceps tendon in the cubital fossa
- ❑ E is overlain by the pronator teres muscle
- ❑ F is larger than the ulnar artery

2.58 Abdominal aortic aneurysm

- ❑ A may cause embolisation to lower limbs
- ❑ B is more common in males
- ❑ C can almost always be treated by endovascular stenting
- ❑ D can be detected by screening
- ❑ E should be operated upon when it is 5.5 cm long

2.59 In coronary artery bypass surgery

- ❑ A the patency rate of internal mammary artery grafts is approximately 90% at 10 years
- ❑ B the patency rate of vein grafts is approximately 80% at 10 years
- ❑ C the main risk factor predictive of outcome is left atrial function
- ❑ D early failure of the internal mammary graft function is usually due to a technical problem
- ❑ E long-term failure of vein grafts is due to suture fragmentation with embolisation

2.60 Glomus tumours

- ❑ A are derived from the Schwann cells
- ❑ B only occur under the finger or toe nails
- ❑ C typically give rise to paroxysms of severe pain
- ❑ D have a malignant potential
- ❑ E are typically palpable

2.61 Nitric oxide

- ❑ A causes platelet aggregation
- ❑ B causes relaxation of smooth muscle
- ❑ C uptake is increased by endotoxins
- ❑ D diffuses freely between cells
- ❑ E causes vasodilatation

2.62 In the diabetic foot

- ❑ A ulcers are usually painful
- ❑ B sensory loss occurs in a stocking distribution
- ❑ C ankle brachial Doppler pressure index may be high
- ❑ D is associated with Charcot joints
- ❑ E amputations are commonplace

2.63 When an arteriovenous fistula is constructed between the radial artery and cephalic vein

- ❑ A the fistula becomes a low-resistance pathway for blood flow
- ❑ B blood flow in the proximal radial artery increases
- ❑ C arterial pressure distal to the fistula will be reduced
- ❑ D the proximal artery elongates and distends with time

2.64 Boundaries of the femoral triangle include

- ❑ A inguinal ligament
- ❑ B adductor longus
- ❑ C adductor magnus
- ❑ D pectineus
- ❑ E iliopsoas

2.65 When treating ulcers on the leg it should be noted that

- ❑ A the annual UK expenditure on ulcer treatment is £20 million
- ❑ B 30% of venous ulcers have a demonstrable arterial component
- ❑ C rolled irregular edges are typical of a venous ulcer
- ❑ D arterial ulcers are usually painful
- ❑ E bacterial colonisation of the ulcer is an indication for topical antibiotics

2.66 Abdominal aortic aneurysm (AAA)

- ❑ A is 4 times more common in males
- ❑ B incidence is falling in Western countries
- ❑ C may be safely observed if asymptomatic and <6 cm in size
- ❑ D is rarely amenable to endoluminal stenting
- ❑ E is less common than popliteal artery aneurysms

2.67 Theme: Carotid artery disease

A Carotid angiography
B MRI head
C CT head
D Right carotid endarterectomy
E Carotid duplex

For each of the patients described below, select the most likely intervention from the list of options above. Each option may be used once, more than once, or not at all.

❑ **1.** A patient has a resolving right-sided CVA. A carotid duplex shows 99% stenosis of the left internal carotid artery and a completely occluded right internal carotid artery.

❑ **2.** A 30-year-old patient with optic neuritis develops a foot drop.

❑ **3.** A resolving recent left-sided hemiparesis with 90% right internal carotid artery stenosis.

2.68 Theme: Varicose veins

A Varicose vein surgery
B IV heparin
C Elevation and NSAIDs
D Compression and warfarin

For each of the patients described below, select the most likely intervention from the list of options above. Each option may be used once, more than once, or not at all.

❑ **1.** A 54-year-old man presents with varicose veins and a bleeding varicose ulcer.

❑ **2.** A 30-year-old woman presents with varicose veins and an acute episode of thrombophlebitis.

❑ **3.** A 45-year-old woman presents with varicose veins and a swollen leg. Duplex confirms a DVT.

2.69 Theme: Lower limb ischaemia

A Surgical embolectomy
B Femoropopliteal bypass graft
C Angioplasty
D Correct the risk factors and provide conservative treatment
E Aortofemoral bypass graft

Select the most appropriate option above for the treatment of the patients below. Each option may be used once, more than once, or not at all.

❑ **1.** A 55-year-old man presents with a sudden onset of severe pain in his left foot and calf. There is no preceding history of intermittent claudication but he experienced a myocardial infarction 2 weeks ago. He is unable to move his foot, which is now mottled and cold. There are absent pulses below his left knee but a palpable femoral pulsation. ECG reveals Q waves with sinus rhythm.

❑ **2.** A 75-year-old man presents to the outpatient clinic with right buttock and thigh pain when walking 100 yards. He smokes 30 cigarettes per day and has a poor cardiac history (3 previous MI, hypertension and left ventricular failure). Ankle brachial Doppler pressure ratio in the right leg is 0.3 and that on the left 0.6. An arteriogram shows an isolated 3 cm 80% stenosis in the right common iliac artery with good run-off. There is evidence of 40% stenosis in the left superficial femoral artery with well-developed collaterals.

❑ **3.** A 65-year-old man presents with pain in his foot when at rest. He has given up smoking and is otherwise fit and well. Angiography shows a 10 cm block in the superficial femoral artery with good distal run-off.

CHAPTER 3: HEAD, NECK, ENDOCRINE AND PAEDIATRIC

3.1 Structures related to the superficial part of the submandibular gland include

- ❑ A platysma
- ❑ B mandibular branch of the facial nerve
- ❑ C facial artery
- ❑ D facial vein
- ❑ E deep cervical fascia

3.2 Theme: Anatomy of joints in the head and neck

A Atlanto-occipital
B Temporomandibular
C Intervertebral disc
D Cricothyroid
E Coronal suture
F Cricoarytenoid
G Atlantoaxial

For each of the statements below, select the most likely joint from the list above. Each option may be used once, more than once, or not at all.

❑ **1.** Has a fibrocartilagenous intra-articular disc.

❑ **2.** Is stabilised by a transverse ligament.

❑ **3.** Is a saddle joint.

3.3 The posterior tongue contains

- ❑ A vallate papillae
- ❑ B lymphoid tissue
- ❑ C filiform papillae
- ❑ D fungiform papillae

3.4 In axillary lymph node dissection

- ❑ A the medial wall of the axilla is formed by the serratus anterior
- ❑ B the clavipectoral fascia on the edge of the pectoralis major should be divided to enter the axilla
- ❑ C inadvertent division of the thoracodorsal nerve may lead to a winged scapula
- ❑ D level II nodes are those lying lateral to pectoralis minor
- ❑ E an anaesthetic patch on the upper medial arm is a recognised complication

3.5 Surgical anatomy of the thyroid

- ❑ A the superior thyroid artery enters the upper pole of the thyroid gland close to the recurrent laryngeal nerve
- ❑ B damage to the external laryngeal nerve causes loss of high-pitched phonation
- ❑ C the inferior thyroid artery arises from the origin of the external carotid artery
- ❑ D the inferior thyroid artery should be ligated as far laterally as possible
- ❑ E the isthmus lies anterior to the trachea

3.6 The thyroid gland

- ❑ A initially moves down on swallowing
- ❑ B lies superficial to the myofascial layer in the neck
- ❑ C receives 5% of the total cardiac output
- ❑ D derives its arterial supply solely from branches of the external carotid
- ❑ E has a venous plexus draining into the internal jugular and brachiocephalic veins

3.7 The Eustachian tube

- ❑ A connects the middle ear and oropharynx
- ❑ B opens by the palatine tonsil
- ❑ C has a bony origin in the sphenoid bone
- ❑ D has a cartilaginous anterior part
- ❑ E is more horizontal in the child

3.8 The tongue

- ❑ A receives sensory innervation from the vagus nerve
- ❑ B protrudes to the side of a unilateral lower motor nerve lesion
- ❑ C is active during the voluntary phase of swallowing
- ❑ D is retracted by the hyoglossus muscle
- ❑ E contains lymphoid tissue
- ❑ F has intrinsic muscles that are not attached to any bone

3.9 The parotid gland

- ❑ A is encapsulated by the investing layer of deep cervical fascia
- ❑ B receives its blood supply directly from the external carotid artery
- ❑ C is traversed by the facial artery
- ❑ D is separated from the carotid sheath by the styloid process
- ❑ E contains the common facial vein
- ❑ F has a duct that passes anteriorly, superficial to the masseter

3.10 The submandibular gland

- ❑ A lies below the digastric muscle
- ❑ B has the hypoglossal nerve running through it
- ❑ C lies both below and above the lower mandible
- ❑ D is superficial to the hyoglossus
- ❑ E has the facial artery running through it

3.11 The true vocal folds are

- ❑ A lined by respiratory epithelium
- ❑ B formed by the lower free edge of the quadrangular membranes
- ❑ C abducted by the lateral cricoarytenoid muscles
- ❑ D abducted by the posterior cricoarytenoid muscles
- ❑ E tensed by contractions of the cricothyroid muscles
- ❑ F innervated by sensory fibres of the internal laryngeal nerves

3.12 The posterior triangle of the neck contains the

- ❑ A great auricular nerve
- ❑ B omohyoid muscle
- ❑ C supraclavicular nerves
- ❑ D roots of the brachial plexus
- ❑ E vertebral artery

3.13 The chorda tympani

- ❑ A contains taste fibres
- ❑ B is secretomotor to the parotid salivary gland
- ❑ C exits the middle ear via the stylomastoid foramen
- ❑ D is vulnerable to damage during parotid surgery
- ❑ E is damaged by compression at the stylomastoid foramen
- ❑ F joins the lingual nerve

3.14 The pituitary fossa

- ❑ A can be seen on a lateral skull X-ray
- ❑ B lies above the sphenoid bone
- ❑ C is associated with the cavernous sinus
- ❑ D lies in the middle cerebral fossa
- ❑ E tumours usually press upon the posterior part of the optic chiasma

3.15 The recurrent laryngeal nerve

- ❑ A supplies all intrinsic laryngeal muscles
- ❑ B supplies the cricothyroid muscle
- ❑ C supplies sensation to the subglottic region
- ❑ D is sensory to the supraglottic region
- ❑ E supplies the sternothyroid muscle

3.16 The middle meatus

- ❑ A drains the nasolacrimal duct
- ❑ B contains the bulla ethmoidalis
- ❑ C drains the sphenoidal air sinus
- ❑ D drains the posterior ethmoidal air sinus
- ❑ E is lined by olfactory epithelium

3.17 Occlusion of the posterior cerebral artery causes

- ❑ A nystagmus
- ❑ B visual disturbances
- ❑ C dysphasia
- ❑ D contralateral hemiplegia
- ❑ E bilateral homonymous hemianopia

3.18 Branchial cysts

- ❑ A pass between the inferior and middle constrictors
- ❑ B contain cholesterol crystals
- ❑ C frequently become infected
- ❑ D may present in childhood

3.19 Parotid adenoma

- ❑ A is the commonest salivary neoplasm
- ❑ B is found in the deep and superficial part of the gland
- ❑ C characteristically produces a facial nerve palsy
- ❑ D is more common in males
- ❑ E Frey's syndrome is an associated complication of parotid surgery

3.20 Theme: Laryngeal cancer

A Total laryngectomy and neck dissection
B Radiotherapy
C Chemotherapy
D Hemilaryngectomy (vertical)
E Supraglottic laryngectomy (horizontal) and neck dissection
F Excision of vocal cord mucosa

For each of the patients below, select the most likely single treatment from the options listed above. Each option may be used once, more than once, or not at all.

❑ **1.** A 50-year-old man presents with a hoarse voice. Clinical examination and investigations reveal a small invasive carcinoma of the right vocal cord. The right vocal cord is paralysed and there is a 4-cm lymph node in the right anterior neck.

❑ **2.** A 65-year-old man is found to have a T_1 carcinoma of the vocal cord. There is no involvement of the anterior commissure.

❑ **3.** A 60-year-old woman is found to have a carcinoma in situ of the left vocal cord.

❑ **4.** A 55-year-old woman is found to have a glottic carcinoma involving the anterior commissure.

❑ **5.** A 70-year-old woman has a large supraglottic carcinoma.

3.21 Theme: Lumps in the neck

A Cystic hygroma
B Carotid body tumour
C Sternocleidomastoid muscle tumour
D Branchial cyst
E Cervical lymphadenopathy
F Thyroid adenoma
G Carotid artery aneurysm

For each of the patients below, choose the most appropriate diagnosis from the list above. Each answer may be used once, more than once, or not at all.

❑ **1.** A 3-year-old child has a slow-growing, painless swelling at the right side of the base of the neck. Examination revealed a fluctuant swelling which transilluminates.

❑ **2.** A 32-year-old woman complained of a swelling situated between the anterior and posterior triangles of the neck on the anterior surface of the upper half of the sternomastoid muscle that had been present for the past week. It was painless on examination. She gave a history of a similar swelling a few months ago which regressed spontaneously.

❑ **3.** A 35-year-old woman has had a painless swelling in the posterior triangle of her neck for 2 months. She works as an animal handler.

3.22 Maxillary sinus carcinoma

❑ A may cause anosmia
❑ B may be caused by the long-term presence of a foreign body
❑ C may cause trismus
❑ D may cause numbness of the face
❑ E metastasise to lymph nodes

3.23 Anatomy of the orbit

❑ A the supraorbital nerve passes through the superorbital fissure
❑ B the ophthalmic artery passes through the supraorbital fissure
❑ C the optic nerve is surrounded by pia, arachnoid and dura mater
❑ D the frontal nerve passes through the tendinous membrane
❑ E the nasociliary nerve supplies the cornea
❑ F sectioning of the inferior ramus of the oculomotor nerve will produce a ptosis
❑ G the ophthalmic artery is a branch of the internal carotid artery

3.24 The following are characteristic of a malignant thyroid nodule:

❑ A Horner's syndrome
❑ B cystic degeneration on ultrasound
❑ C deviation of the trachea
❑ D dysphagia
❑ E stridor
❑ F thyrotoxicosis

3.25 The salivary glands

❑ A secrete >1000 ml/day
❑ B produce saliva which has about the same pH as plasma
❑ C secrete amylase
❑ D produce secretions which contain a higher molar concentration of potassium compared with plasma
❑ E produce hypertonic secretions

3.26 Theme: Congenital neck lumps

A Laryngocele
B Thyroglossal cyst
C Branchial cyst
D Desmoid cyst
E Dermoid cyst
F Lymphangioma
G Chemodectoma

For each of the patients below, chose the most appropriate diagnosis from those above. Each may be used once, more than once, or not at all.

❑ **1.** A 55-year-old man presents with a long-standing history of mild stridor and hoarseness which suddenly deteriorates. A large soft swelling over the thyrohyoid membrane is felt on palpation. The swelling disappears when pressure is applied.

❑ **2.** A 7-year-old girl presents with a painless cystic swelling anterior to the thyroid cartilage. The swelling is transilluminable, mobile in the lateral direction and moves on swallowing.

3.27 Glue ear is associated with

❑ A enlarged pharyngeal tonsils
❑ B cleft palate
❑ C Eustachian tube dysfunction
❑ D otosclerosis

3.28 Piriform fossa tumours

❑ A are usually columnar epithelium in origin
❑ B cannot be seen using indirect laryngoscopy
❑ C may cause pain referred to the ear
❑ D drain to the deep cervical nodes

3.29 Pain in the ear during acute tonsillitis is due to the

❑ A superior laryngeal nerve
❑ B glossopharyngeal nerve
❑ C facial nerve
❑ D hypoglossal nerve
❑ E lesser palatine nerve

3.30 In the use of eye drops

❑ A timolol reduces intraocular pressure
❑ B adrenaline increases intraocular pressure
❑ C pilocarpine decreases intraocular pressure
❑ D tetracaine (amethocaine) constricts the pupil
❑ E morphine dilates the pupil

3.31 Infarction of the left occipital lobe would produce

❑ A left homonymous hemianopia
❑ B right visual field loss
❑ C macular sparing
❑ D blindness in the right eye
❑ E paralysis of the lateral rectus muscle

3.32 Bilateral vocal cord paralysis

❑ A is a recognised sequela of diphtheria infection
❑ B after thyroid surgery may require intubation
❑ C is treated with arytenoidectomy
❑ D is caused by superior laryngeal nerve injury

3.33 Tracheostomy

❑ A reduces the respiratory dead space in an adult by approximately 70 ml
❑ B may produce a supraglottic stenosis
❑ C tube changing should be avoided for 3 days postoperatively
❑ D is usually performed through the third and fourth tracheal rings
❑ E tube dislodgement may produce erosion of the innominate artery

3.34 Recognised complications of tracheostomy include

❑ A surgical emphysema
❑ B pneumonia
❑ C air embolism
❑ D haemorrhage
❑ E subglottic stenosis

3.35 Complications of submandibular gland excision include

❑ A weakness of the angle of the mouth
❑ B anaesthesia of the contralateral half of the tongue
❑ C deviation of the tongue to the contralateral side
❑ D Frey's syndrome
❑ E damage to the retromandibular vein

3.36 Parotid gland tumours

❑ A account for approximately 80% of all salivary gland tumours
❑ B are most commonly benign
❑ C are always slow growing
❑ D can present with otalgia
❑ E can be core biopsied safely with MRI

3.37 Theme: Thyroid disease

A Hot nodule in the thyroid gland
B Recurrent thyroid lymphoma
C Follicular adenoma
D Early anaplastic carcinoma
E Follicular carcinoma

For each of the thyroid conditions above, select the most appropriate treatment or description. Each option may be used once, more than once, or not at all.

❑ **1.** A combination of radiotherapy and chemotherapy is a suitable treatment for this.

❑ **2.** A combination of resection and radiotherapy is a suitable treatment for this.

❑ **3.** Occurs in Plummer's syndrome.

❑ **4.** Thyroid lobectomy only is a suitable treatment.

❑ **5.** A combination of total thyroidectomy and radio-iodine is a suitable treatment for this.

3.38 Ludwig's angina

- ❑ A is usually caused by an infected tooth
- ❑ B may cause dysphagia
- ❑ C should be regarded as a surgical emergency
- ❑ D is treated with oral amoxicillin
- ❑ E is caused by peptostreptococci

3.39 Oral cavity cancer

- ❑ A has no gender predilection
- ❑ B is most commonly found on the anterior two-thirds of the tongue
- ❑ C rarely presents with pain
- ❑ D responds well to chemotherapy
- ❑ E should be treated with surgery if bony invasion occurs

3.40 Transection of the anterior division of the mandibular nerve (Vc) in the infratemporal fossa results in

- ❑ A ipsilateral paralysis of the buccinator muscle
- ❑ B dysphagia
- ❑ C ipsilateral anaesthesia of the mandibular teeth
- ❑ D deviation of the jaw to the side of the lesion on protrusion
- ❑ E ipsilateral anaesthesia of the mucosa of the oral vestibule

3.41 Epistaxis

- ❑ A usually arises from the posteromedial nasal septum
- ❑ B can be controlled by placement of a Fogarty balloon catheter
- ❑ C may be a presentation of leukaemia
- ❑ D may require ligation of the maxillary artery
- ❑ E is best treated by bedrest and sedation

3.42 Lateral swellings of the neck include

- ❑ A cervical ribs
- ❑ B thyroglossal cysts
- ❑ C pharyngeal pouches
- ❑ D carotid body tumours (chemodectomas)
- ❑ E laryngoceles

3.43 Acute otitis media

- ❑ A is often accompanied by a purulent discharge from the ear
- ❑ B is usually caused by *Escherichia coli*
- ❑ C rarely causes constitutional upset in children
- ❑ D invariably forms a cholesteatoma if resolution does not occur by 6 weeks
- ❑ E is primarily treated with myringotomy

3.44 On turning the head to the left

- ❑ A the left sternocleidomastoid muscle is the main agonist
- ❑ B movement takes place at the atlanto-occipital joint
- ❑ C neural impulses pass via the spinal accessory nerve
- ❑ D the axis of rotation runs vertically through the odontoid process
- ❑ E movement is limited typically by cervical vertebrae

3.45 Within the orbit

- ❑ A the optic nerve is invested by meninges
- ❑ B ischaemic necrosis of the retina follows optic nerve transection
- ❑ C blow-out fractures can cause diplopia
- ❑ D trochlear nerve lesions cause ptosis
- ❑ E frontal nerve lesions depress the corneal reflex

3.46 Salivary gland calculi

- ❑ A usually arise in the parotid gland
- ❑ B are most commonly found in the sixth decade of life
- ❑ C are associated with a more alkaline saliva
- ❑ D are more common in diabetics
- ❑ E are mostly visible on plain X-ray

3.47 Complications of otitis media include

- ❑ A papilloedema
- ❑ B facial nerve paralysis
- ❑ C cerebellar abscess
- ❑ D homonymous hemianopia
- ❑ E sudden deafness

3.48 A Le Fort-III maxillary fracture

- ❑ A is usually treated conservatively
- ❑ B involves the lateral wall of the orbit
- ❑ C rarely results in malocclusion
- ❑ D may cause gross mid-facial swelling
- ❑ E involves the ethmoidal bone

3.49 Midline swellings of the neck include

- ❑ A cystic hygromas
- ❑ B plunging ranulas
- ❑ C subhyoid bursas
- ❑ D branchial cysts
- ❑ E arteriovenous fistulas

3.50 Typical presenting features of intracranial tumours include

- ❑ A nocturnal headache exacerbated by coughing
- ❑ B mood changes
- ❑ C diplopia on lateral gaze
- ❑ D apnoeic attacks
- ❑ E vomiting

3.51 Papillary carcinoma of the thyroid

- ❑ A has a strong association with previous radiation exposure
- ❑ B secretes calcitonin
- ❑ C is found in iodine-poor areas
- ❑ D is frequently multifocal
- ❑ E usually presents with distant metastases
- ❑ F is treated with thyroxine following total thyroidectomy to suppress TSH levels
- ❑ G is a disease of the elderly

3.52 The following are causes of respiratory distress following thyroidectomy:

- ❑ A unilateral recurrent laryngeal nerve section
- ❑ B aspiration
- ❑ C laryngeal oedema
- ❑ D hypocalcaemia
- ❑ E tracheomalacia

3.53 Laryngeal carcinoma

- ❑ A has an equal sex incidence
- ❑ B is most commonly supraglottic
- ❑ C usually presents with stridor
- ❑ D is radioresistant
- ❑ E should be assessed by microlaryngoscopy in difficult cases

3.54 Structures superficial to the sternocleidomastoid include the

- ❑ A transverse cervical nerve
- ❑ B transverse cervical artery
- ❑ C great auricular nerve
- ❑ D external jugular vein
- ❑ E inferior thyroid artery

3.55 The inferior thyroid artery

- ❑ A supplies the inferior and superior parathyroid glands
- ❑ B supplies the oesophagus
- ❑ C arises from the external carotid artery
- ❑ D is ligated close to the gland in a thyroidectomy
- ❑ E supplies the inferior pole of the thyroid

3.56 Structures passing through the foramen magnum include

- ❑ A medulla oblongata
- ❑ B vertebral arteries
- ❑ C spinal arteries
- ❑ D vertebral veins
- ❑ E dura mater

3.57 The internal jugular veins

- ❑ A emerge from the posterior compartment of the jugular foramen
- ❑ B drain the cavernous venous sinus
- ❑ C have the ansa cervicalis as an anterior relation
- ❑ D are the most anterior structures in the carotid sheath
- ❑ E drain into the brachiocephalic veins behind the sternoclavicular joints
- ❑ F lie deep to the sternocleidomastoid

3.58 The superior vena cava

- ❑ A has a valve at its entry into the left atrium
- ❑ B drains only the head, neck and upper body
- ❑ C receives the thoracic duct
- ❑ D ends behind the second costal cartilage
- ❑ E enters the heart at the level of the sternal angle

3.59 The ophthalmic artery

- ❑ A has the central artery of the retina as its terminal branch
- ❑ B supplies both the anterior and posterior ethmoidal arteries
- ❑ C originates from the internal carotid artery
- ❑ D enters the orbit through the superior orbital fissure
- ❑ E supplies the skin over the forehead
- ❑ F travels with the nasociliary nerve
- ❑ G supplies the cornea

3.60 The external carotid artery

- ❑ A terminates at the level of the cricoid cartilage
- ❑ B is crossed by the posterior belly of the digastric muscle
- ❑ C lies superficial to the hypoglossal nerve
- ❑ D is separated from the internal carotid artery by the stylopharyngeus and styloglossus muscles
- ❑ E contains the carotid sinus

3.61 The spinal canal (vertebral foramen) is

- ❑ A anterior to the ligamentum flavum
- ❑ B posterior to the vertebral disc
- ❑ C constant in diameter
- ❑ D lateral to the facets
- ❑ E ends at L1

3.62 The thoracic duct

- ❑ A lies to the right of the aorta
- ❑ B opens into the superior vena cava
- ❑ C is anterior to the left subclavian artery
- ❑ D commences at the level of T10
- ❑ E drains into the right subclavian vein

3.63 Pharyngeal pouch

❑ A is common in boys under 6 years of age
❑ B commonly presents with aspiration
❑ C can be treated by myotomy alone
❑ D should be investigated by endoscopy
❑ E is more common on the right side

3.64 Pharyngeal web is associated with

❑ A megaloblastic anaemia
❑ B carcinoma
❑ C Plummer–Vinson syndrome
❑ D female gender
❑ E recurrent pneumonia

3.65 Theme: Calcium metabolism

A Primary hyperparathyroidism
B Secondary hyperparathyroidism
C Tertiary hyperparathyroidism
D Parathyroid hormone
E Hypoparathyroidism

For each of the points below, select the most appropriate answer from the list above. Each option may be used once, more than once, or not at all.

❑ **1.** Is associated with a normal serum calcium.

❑ **2.** Is usually caused by an adenoma.

❑ **3.** Is produced by renal disease.

❑ **4.** Is caused by thyroid surgery.

3.66 Theme: Treatment of thyrotoxicosis

A Propranolol
B Carbimazole
C Radio-iodine
D Subtotal thyroidectomy
E Total thyroidectomy

For each of the patients described below, select the most likely treatment from the list of options above. Each option may be used once, more than once, or not at all.

❑ **1.** A teenager presents with symptoms and signs of thyrotoxicosis.

❑ **2.** A 65-year-old presents with a CVA and atrial fibrillation due to hyperthyroidism.

❑ **3.** Medical treatment has failed to cure a patient with thyrotoxicosis.

3.67 Theme: Familial endocrine disease

A MEN-1 syndrome
B MEN-2 syndrome
C Phaeochromocytoma
D Papillary carcinoma of the thyroid
E Hyperparathyroidism
F Diabetes

For each of the statements below select the most likely answer from the list above. Each option may be used once, more than once, or not at all.

❑ **1.** Is an autosomal dominant condition with high penetrance.

❑ **2.** Presents with tumours of the anterior pituitary, parathyroids and pancreatic islets.

❑ **3.** Is the most common presenting lesion in MEN-1 syndrome.

3.68 Causes of hypercalcaemia include

- ❑ A Addison's disease
- ❑ B renal failure
- ❑ C diabetes mellitus
- ❑ D sarcoidosis
- ❑ E thyrotoxicosis

3.69 Theme: Paediatric investigations

A A 'double-bubble sign' on plain abdominal X-ray (AXR)
B A 'cone' on contrast enema
C Hypochloraemic metabolic alkalosis
D Intramural gas on plain AXR
E Air-filled cysts in the left chest
F A 'target' lesion on abdominal ultrasound
G A type-II curve on a diuretic renogram
H Clubbed renal calyces on a micturating cystogram

For each of the clinical scenarios below, select the most appropriate feature on investigation from the list above. Each option may be used once, more than once, or not at all.

❑ **1.** A 10-hour-old term baby presents with persistent non-bile-stained vomiting.

❑ **2.** A 10-day-old baby, born at 30 weeks, presents with bile-stained vomiting and bloody diarrhoea.

❑ **3.** An 8-month-old infant presents with colicky abdominal pain and bleeding per rectum.

❑ **4.** A 2-day-old baby presents with abdominal distension, bile-stained vomiting and failure to pass meconium.

3.70 Fontanelles of the skull

- ❑ A early fontanelle closure is associated with microcephaly
- ❑ B allow for brain growth
- ❑ C the anterior fontanelle is larger than the posterior fontanelle
- ❑ D the anterior fontanelle lies on the anterior sagittal plane
- ❑ E the posterior fontanelle can be used to obtain blood samples from the sagittal sinus in the midline

3.71 Common causes of unilateral nasal discharge in children include

- ❑ A cystic fibrosis
- ❑ B nasal polyps
- ❑ C foreign body
- ❑ D common cold
- ❑ E nasopharyngeal carcinoma

3.72 Cleft lip

- ❑ A affects boys more than girls
- ❑ B affects 1 in 750 live births
- ❑ C has a declining incidence
- ❑ D is associated with palate defects in 50% of cases
- ❑ E has a 25% subsequent increased risk following a previous affected child

3.73 Inguinal hernia in children

- ❑ A usually presents with strangulation
- ❑ B frequently becomes irreducible in the first 3 months of life
- ❑ C requires inguinal herniorrhaphy in most cases
- ❑ D should be repaired after 1 year of age
- ❑ E should be repaired without delivering the testicle into the wound
- ❑ F may contain ovary

3.74 Intussusception

- ❑ A usually presents between the ages of 2 and 3 years
- ❑ B is ileocolic in the majority of cases
- ❑ C is usually found to have an anatomical cause
- ❑ D may be associated with a viral illness
- ❑ E may present with screaming attacks

3.75 The Eustachian tube in the infant

- ❑ A connects the middle ear to the oropharynx
- ❑ B opens by the palatine tonsil
- ❑ C has a bony portion in the sphenoid bone
- ❑ D has a cartilaginous medial segment
- ❑ E is more horizontal in the child

3.76 Neonates

- ❑ A can concentrate urine to 1400 mOsm/l
- ❑ B weighing 3 kg have a blood volume of 450 ml
- ❑ C should be operated in theatres with an ambient temperature of 20 °C
- ❑ D often are unable to tolerate oral feeds following major bowel surgery
- ❑ E should have a recommended oral feed of 350 ml/kg per day in the first week of life

3.77 Cystic fibrosis

- ❑ A is the commonest autosomal recessive condition in white people
- ❑ B may present with intestinal obstruction
- ❑ C patients have an increased risk of developing pancreatic tumours
- ❑ D is associated with nasal polyps
- ❑ E only presents in children

3.78 An undescended testicle

- ❑ A should be treated with hormones if descent is incomplete at 1 year of age
- ❑ B can be differentiated from a retractile testis by clinical examination
- ❑ C if untreated has a higher risk of torsion
- ❑ D occurs bilaterally in 30% of cases
- ❑ E is treated with LHRH analogues

3.79 Prolactin

- ❑ A secretion decreases after surgery
- ❑ B is under dopaminergic control
- ❑ C secretion increases after trauma
- ❑ D is involved in the secretion of milk during lactation
- ❑ E secretion is under hypothalamic control

3.80 In exomphalos

❑ A there is a 25% mortality rate after birth
❑ B the herniated organs are covered by a membrane derived from the umbilical cord
❑ C there is an association with trisomy 13
❑ D the liver is rarely involved
❑ E bowel can be inadvertently damaged by the cord clamp

3.81 Congenital hypertrophic pyloric stenosis

❑ A typically presents at birth
❑ B is more common in males
❑ C may result in hypocalcaemia
❑ D may result in a metabolic alkalosis
❑ E is best investigated by contrast examination

3.82 Abdominal pain in a 4-year-old girl can be the presenting feature of

❑ A pneumonia
❑ B intussusception
❑ C meningitis
❑ D viral infection
❑ E intestinal atresia

3.83 Undescended testis (UDT)

❑ A occurs in 1% of term infants
❑ B will descend in 75% of cases by the first year of life
❑ C placement within the scrotum should be undertaken by 1 year of age
❑ D placement within the scrotum reduces the risk of subsequent tumour development
❑ E is best located with CT scanning when in a suspected intra-abdominal position

3.84 In infantile hypertrophic pyloric stenosis

❑ A there is typically a hyperkalaemic, hyperchloraemic alkalosis
❑ B the diagnosis is usually clinical
❑ C females are more often affected
❑ D jaundice is seen in 10% of children

3.85 Inguinal hernia in infancy

- ❑ A is usually of the direct variety
- ❑ B is more common in babies born prematurely
- ❑ C can safely be left until the child weighs over 10 kg
- ❑ D does not routinely require a herniorrhaphy
- ❑ E is not associated with a patent processus vaginalis

3.86 An infant born at 32 weeks gestation, weighing 1.2 kg

- ❑ A always requires artificial ventilation for 24 hours after birth
- ❑ B has a smaller insensible fluid loss than an adult
- ❑ C may require placement of a central line in the internal jugular vein
- ❑ D is at risk of necrotising enterocolitis
- ❑ E will not develop pyloric stenosis

3.87 Hirschsprung's disease

- ❑ A almost always involves the rectum
- ❑ B can involve the entire intestine
- ❑ C is continuous in its distribution
- ❑ D is characterised by an excess of ganglion cells in the myenteric plexus
- ❑ E may present in adulthood

3.88 Intussusception

- ❑ A is the commonest cause of small bowel obstruction in children under the age of 18 months
- ❑ B classically presents with brick-red coloured stools
- ❑ C is infrequently associated with a pathological lead-point over the age of 18 months
- ❑ D can be treated safely with an air enema
- ❑ E is an unusual cause of unexplained collapse in a child

3.89 Oesophageal atresia

- ❑ A can occur without a tracheo-oesophageal fistula
- ❑ B is rarely associated with other structural abnormalities
- ❑ C definitive repair can be delayed for several months
- ❑ D is associated with maternal polyhydramnios
- ❑ E has an incidence of approximately 1:4000 live births

3.90 Congenital diaphragmatic hernia

- ❑ A is found on the left side in over 75% of cases
- ❑ B can be detected on prenatal ultrasound scanning
- ❑ C should be regarded as a surgical emergency and be repaired immediately
- ❑ D may present late with failure to thrive
- ❑ E is associated with gut malrotation

3.91 Duodenal atresia

- ❑ A is associated with trisomy 21
- ❑ B is corrected by a gastroenterostomy
- ❑ C is not usually obvious on plain AXR
- ❑ D can present at 6 weeks of age

3.92 Hydrocele of infancy

- ❑ A is usually of the 'communicating' variety
- ❑ B should be left until the child is beyond 12 months of age before repair
- ❑ C does not occur in females
- ❑ D cannot be effectively treated by simple division of the patent processus vaginalis
- ❑ E may not surround the testis

3.93 Positions for an ectopic testis include

- ❑ A inguinal
- ❑ B penile
- ❑ C intra-abdominal
- ❑ D femoral
- ❑ E high scrotal

3.94 Hydrocele in a 5-year-old

- ❑ A should be aspirated
- ❑ B will resolve spontaneously
- ❑ C should be operated on via groin incision
- ❑ D can be performed as day-case surgery

CHAPTER 4: ABDOMEN

4.1 Levator ani

- ❑ A forms the roof of the ischiorectal fossa
- ❑ B may be divided into deep and superficial parts
- ❑ C is supplied by L4/L5
- ❑ D origin includes the obturator fascia
- ❑ E lies at the bifurcation of the aorta

4.2 Theme: Surface/radiological anatomy of the anterior abdominal wall

A Transpyloric plane
B L4 vertebral body
C L5 vertebral body
D Mid-inguinal point
E Above and medial to the pubic tubercle
F Sacroiliac joint
G Below and lateral to the pubic tubercle
H Midpoint of inguinal ligament
I Umbilicus
J 12th rib
K 10th rib
L Transtubercular plane

For each of the statements below, select the most likely location of the following from the list above. Each option may be used once, more than once, or not at all.

❑ **1.** Division of the aorta into the common iliac vessels.

❑ **2.** Ureter.

❑ **3.** Femoral artery.

❑ **4.** Upper poles of the kidneys.

4.3 The superior mesenteric artery

- ❑ A supplies the whole of the jejunum and ileum
- ❑ B lies to the left of the superior mesenteric vein
- ❑ C lies behind the neck of the pancreas
- ❑ D lies posterior to the third part of the duodenum
- ❑ E lies above the splenic vein

4.4 Through the epiploic foramen the

- ❑ A caudate lobe of the liver is palpable in the lesser sac
- ❑ B inferior vena cava lies posteriorly
- ❑ C portal vein lies anteriorly
- ❑ D right gastric artery lies posteriorly
- ❑ E second part of the duodenum forms the lower boundary

4.5 Borders of Hesselbach's triangle include

- ❑ A the inferior epigastric artery
- ❑ B the inguinal ligament
- ❑ C the medial border of the rectus abdominis muscle
- ❑ D lacunar ligament
- ❑ E the femoral artery

4.6 The epiploic foramen

- ❑ A has the quadrate lobe of the liver as a superior boundary
- ❑ B has the gastroduodenal artery lying medially
- ❑ C has the portal vein lying posterior
- ❑ D has the third part of the duodenum lying inferiorly
- ❑ E is involved in Pringle's manoeuvre

4.7 The psoas muscle

- ❑ A originates in part from the lumbar transverse processes
- ❑ B inserts into the greater trochanter
- ❑ C flexes the hip joint
- ❑ D externally rotates the leg
- ❑ E is supplied by the femoral nerve

4.8 Theme: Anatomy of abdominal vasculature

A Inferior mesenteric vein
B Superior mesenteric vein
C Left gastric vein
D Right renal artery
E Left renal vein
F Gastroduodenal artery
G Portal vein
H Left suprarenal artery
I Left colic artery
J Ileocolic artery
K Splenic artery
L Middle colic artery
M Superior mesenteric artery
N Left gonadal vein

For each of the statements below, select the most likely option from the list above. Each option may be used once, more than once, or not at all.

❑ **1.** A site of portosystemic anastomosis.

❑ **2.** Lies posterior to the first part of the duodenum.

❑ **3.** Drains into the splenic vein.

❑ **4.** Lies posterior to the inferior vena cava.

4.9 The uterus

❑ A is related to the small bowel
❑ B has the ureters running laterally across it
❑ C is supplied by a direct branch of the external iliac artery
❑ D is covered completely with peritoneum
❑ E is related to pouch of Douglas
❑ F is supplied by the pudendal nerves
❑ G is supplied by the obturator nerves

4.10 The liver

- ❑ A the left lobe is in direct contact with the left suprarenal gland
- ❑ B is covered completely with peritoneum
- ❑ C is attached to the diaphragm by the falciform ligament
- ❑ D is in contact with both the oesophagus and the stomach
- ❑ E the right and left lobes can be divided individually into four vascular segments

4.11 Theme: Anatomy of the viscera and organs in the abdomen

A Suprarenal gland
B Ileum
C Coronary ligament
D Stomach
E Spleen
F Pancreas
G Meckel's diverticulum
H Kidney

For each of the statements below, select the most likely option from the list above. Each option may be used once, more than once, or not at all.

❑ **1.** Is crossed by the inferior mesenteric vein.

❑ **2.** Has a mesentery attached to the pelvic brim.

❑ **3.** May have an umbilical attachment.

❑ **4.** Lies in the lienorenal ligament.

❑ **5.** Has veins forming portosystemic anastomoses.

4.12 The inferior mesenteric vein

- ❑ A drains the rectum
- ❑ B lies anterior to the left renal vein
- ❑ C is a tributary of the portal vein
- ❑ D lies to the right of the inferior mesenteric artery
- ❑ E lies anterior to the left ureter
- ❑ F drains the ileum

4.13 The portal vein

- ❑ A is anterior to the first part of the duodenum
- ❑ B is formed in the confluence of the superior mesenteric and splenic veins
- ❑ C lies behind the epiploic foramen
- ❑ D receives tributaries from the pancreatic neck
- ❑ E lies partly in the lesser omentum

4.14 Direct branches of the coeliac plexus include the

- ❑ A splenic artery
- ❑ B hepatic artery
- ❑ C superior pancreaticoduodenal artery
- ❑ D right gastric artery
- ❑ E gastroduodenal artery

4.15 The inferior vena cava

- ❑ A carries most of the blood below the diaphragm back to the heart
- ❑ B has the right sympathetic trunk lying behind its right margin
- ❑ C receives direct tributaries from both suprarenal glands
- ❑ D receives direct tributaries from both kidneys
- ❑ E receives direct tributaries from both gonads
- ❑ F is valveless

4.16 Portal vein thrombosis may

- ❑ A occur in patients with thrombophilia
- ❑ B occur after severe appendicitis
- ❑ C cause small bowel infarction
- ❑ D cause small intestinal varicosities
- ❑ E cause splenomegaly

4.17 The internal iliac artery supplies the

- ❑ A sigmoid colon
- ❑ B spinal cord
- ❑ C trochanteric anastomosis
- ❑ D bladder
- ❑ E anterior superior iliac spine anastomosis

4.18 Inguinal lymph nodes receive drainage from the

- ❑ A scrotum
- ❑ B testis
- ❑ C cervix
- ❑ D lumbosacral skin
- ❑ E fallopian tubes

4.19 The superficial inguinal lymph nodes drain the

- ❑ A skin of the gluteal region
- ❑ B skin of the perianal region
- ❑ C uterus
- ❑ D testis
- ❑ E skin of the dorsum of the foot

4.20 Theme: Anatomy of the posterior abdominal wall

A Kidney
B Psoas major muscle
C Lumbar plexus
D Ureter
E Sympathetic trunk
F Ilioinguinal nerve
G Bare area of the liver
H Superior rectal artery

For each of the statements below, select the most likely option from the list above. Each option may be used once, more than once, or not at all.

❑ **1.** Tracts pus to the femoral triangle.

❑ **2.** Lies in the root of the sigmoid mesentery.

❑ **3.** Lies behind the aorta.

❑ **4.** Lies behind the kidney.

4.21 Femoral hernia

❑ A has a high risk of strangulation
❑ B is easily missed in the obese
❑ C is equally common in males and females
❑ D has a neck lying at the level of the inguinal ligament
❑ E may be revealed by scrotal skin invagination

4.22 In gallstone disease

❑ A approximately 50% of patients are symptomatic
❑ B the pain of biliary colic is due to gallbladder ischaemia resulting from temporary cystic duct obstruction
❑ C a mucocele of the gallbladder characteristically contains infected bile
❑ D acute cholecystitis is often associated with gallbladder mucosal ulceration
❑ E an empyema of the gallbladder may cause septic shock
❑ F acute cholecystitis infrequently perforates

4.23 Solitary rectal ulcer syndrome

❑ A usually produces bright-red rectal bleeding
❑ B is associated with excessive passage of mucus
❑ C symptoms are due to repeated anal dilatation
❑ D rectal biopsies show palisading basal cells
❑ E is best treated by excision of the ulcer

4.24 Indications for surgery in ulcerative colitis include

❑ A failure of a significant response to medical treatment of a severe flare after 48 hours
❑ B acute toxic megacolon
❑ C failure of adequate medical treatment of chronic disease over a prolonged period
❑ D the presence of confirmed mild dysplasia on colonic biopsies
❑ E total colitis

4.25 Treatment of small bowel embolus includes

- ❑ A anticoagulation
- ❑ B embolectomy through the femoral artery
- ❑ C digoxin
- ❑ D small bowel resection

4.26 Theme: Abdominal disease

A Intussusception
B Meckel's diverticulum
C Mesenteric ischaemia
D Crohn's disease
E Coeliac disease
F Appendix mass
G Caecal carcinoma

For each of the patients below, select the most likely diagnosis from the list above. Each option may be used once, more than once, or not at all.

❑ **1.** An 80-year-old lady with atrial fibrillation has a 4-day history of abdominal pain and some bleeding rectally.

❑ **2.** A 16-year-old boy presents with a 6-month history of diarrhoea, vomiting and vague right iliac fossa mass. He has a microcytic anaemia.

❑ **3.** An 18-year-old girl presents with a 4-day history of pain in the right iliac fossa, a temperature of 38 °C and diarrhoea.

4.27 Complications of laparoscopic surgery include

- ❑ A surgical emphysema
- ❑ B nitric oxide embolus
- ❑ C pneumothorax
- ❑ D trocar injuries to the iliac artery
- ❑ E deep vein thrombosis

4.28 The following should be considered for colorectal carcinoma screening:

- ❑ A the brother of a patient with familial adenomatous polyposis
- ❑ B a patient with long-standing ulcerative colitis
- ❑ C a patient with long-standing Peutz–Jeghers' syndrome
- ❑ D a patient with Gardner's syndrome
- ❑ E a patient with long-standing diverticular disease

4.29 In Crohn's disease

- ❑ A bowel should be resected back to microscopically normal bowel to prevent recurrence
- ❑ B multiple small resections are preferred to multiple stricturoplasties for multiple, short-segment, small bowel strictures
- ❑ C if proctocolectomy is indicated, rectal excision should preserve perirectal tissues
- ❑ D perianal abscesses are managed with antibiotics

4.30 Colon cancer

- ❑ A is the commonest cause of death due to malignancy in the UK
- ❑ B has a slight female predominance
- ❑ C causes hepatic metastases in 30% of cases at the time of presentation
- ❑ D has an equal incidence in developed and developing countries
- ❑ E has an increasing relative incidence in the right colon in developed countries

4.31 Early poor prognostic factors for acute pancreatitis include

- ❑ A a serum amylase level of >2000 IU
- ❑ B a blood glucose concentration of >6 mmol/l
- ❑ C a serum calcium concentration of <2.4 mmol/l
- ❑ D WCC $>15 \times 10^9$/l
- ❑ E pO_2 <8 kPa
- ❑ F blood urea >10 mmol/l despite adequate fluid replacement
- ❑ G haemoglobin <10 g/dl

4.32 Theme: Abdominal pain investigations

A FBC
B Urea
C Erect chest X-ray
D Supine abdominal X-ray
E ECG
F Mesenteric angiography
G CT abdomen

For each of the patients below, select the most likely diagnostic investigation from the list above. Each option may be used once, more than once, or not at all.

❑ **1.** An 18-year-old man presents with 24 hours of generalised abdominal pain, which has now shifted to the right iliac fossa.

❑ **2.** A 59-year-old woman with a history of rheumatoid arthritis treated with NSAIDs, gold and steroids, presents with 4 hours of acute abdominal pain. This was made worse by the ambulance ride.

❑ **3.** An 85-year-old woman presents with profuse, fresh, red rectal bleeding. She is hypotensive, with a fast irregular pulse.

❑ **4.** A 62-year-old woman is admitted with vomiting, colicky abdominal pain and a distended abdomen. She has previously undergone multiple gynaecological operations.

4.33 Typical endoscopic features of Crohn's disease include

❑ A aphthous ulceration
❑ B pseudomembranes
❑ C loss of the normal vascular pattern
❑ D deep fissuring ulceration with a cobblestone appearance
❑ E microadenomas

4.34 Typical radiological features of acute ulcerative colitis on plain AXR include

❑ A loss of haustrations
❑ B mucosal irregularity
❑ C left-sided faecal loading
❑ D the 'beak' sign
❑ E absence of faecal residue within the actively inflamed part of the colon

4.35 Carcinoid syndrome

❑ A generally produces paroxysmal flushing of the face and trunk
❑ B flushing that may be precipitated by alcohol
❑ C has been shown to respond to octreotide
❑ D does not respond to tumour debulking
❑ E is associated with diarrhoea

4.36 In investigations for inflammatory bowel disease

❑ A endoscopic visual appearances alone usually allow a definitive diagnosis between ulcerative colitis and Crohn's disease
❑ B a barium enema may produce a characteristic lead-pipe appearance
❑ C mucosal granularity on an 'instant' enema suggests at least mild inflammation
❑ D colonoscopy during a disease flare is associated with an increased risk of perforation
❑ E proximal colonic stool on plain AXR in a patient with ulcerative colitis suggests that the proximal large bowel is significantly inflamed

4.37 In colonic polyps

❑ A the incidence of invasive cancer in colonic polyps <1 cm in size is approximately 10%
❑ B the incidence of invasive cancer in colonic polyps 1–2 cm in size is approximately 35%
❑ C the incidence of invasive cancer in colonic polyps >2 cm in size is approximately 80%
❑ D villous adenomas have a greater risk of malignant change than tubular adenomas of the same size

4.38 Epigastric hernias

- ❑ A are often multiple
- ❑ B usually contain small bowel
- ❑ C are frequently irreducible
- ❑ D are often more easily seen than felt
- ❑ E usually require a mesh repair

4.39 Dermatomyositis

- ❑ A is associated with ovarian carcinoma
- ❑ B is associated with breast carcinoma
- ❑ C may precede the development of a malignancy by 5 years
- ❑ D produces a characteristic urticarial rash around the eyelids
- ❑ E improves with treatment of the underlying neoplasm

4.40 Acute acalculous cholecystitis

- ❑ A accounts for approximately 10% of cases of acute cholecystitis
- ❑ B is especially common after colonic surgery
- ❑ C is thought to be related to supersaturation of bile
- ❑ D is commonly seen in patients in the ITU
- ❑ E is diagnosed by full-thickness gallbladder biopsy

4.41 The approximate incidences of Crohn's disease involvement in the gastrointestinal tract are

- ❑ A ileocaecal region only – 40%
- ❑ B colon only – 25%
- ❑ C ileum only – 10%
- ❑ D extensive small bowel disease – 30%
- ❑ E miscellaneous (e.g. confined to the anorectum, oral, gastric areas) – 2%

4.42 Surgical techniques for preserving a traumatised spleen include

- ❑ A omental patch repair
- ❑ B topical thrombogenic agents
- ❑ C wrapping with a Dexon mesh
- ❑ D induced hypotension to minimise haemorrhage
- ❑ E partial splenectomy

4.43 The Child–Pugh classification of hepatocellular function in cirrhosis includes details of

❑ A serum bilirubin
❑ B serum calcium
❑ C white cell count
❑ D core body temperature
❑ E the presence of ascites

4.44 Bile-stained vomiting is a feature of

❑ A mid-gut volvulus
❑ B pyloric stenosis
❑ C intussusception
❑ D oesophageal atresia
❑ E gastro-oesophageal reflux

4.45 Gallstone ileus

❑ A usually follows iatrogenic fistulation of the gallbladder
❑ B is often caused by calculi impacting in the proximal ileum
❑ C often produces complete small bowel obstruction
❑ D may produce air in the biliary tree visible on AXR
❑ E is most common in the <60-year age group

4.46 In the surgical treatment of rectal cancer

❑ A distal intramural spread is often 3 cm
❑ B a distal resection clearance of 5 cm from the rectal tumour is mandatory
❑ C the mesorectum contains an abundance of lymphatic tissue
❑ D irrigation of the divided bowel ends with cytotoxic solutions reduces local tumour recurrence
❑ E exfoliated malignant cells may be found intraluminally, adjacent to resection margins at the time of surgery

4.47 Theme: Abdominal pain investigations – diagnostic

A FBC
B Serum amylase
C Erect chest X-ray
D Supine abdominal X-ray
E Angiography (mesenteric)
F CT
G Barium enema
H Barium meal – small bowel follow-through
I Abdominal ultrasound

For each of the patients described below, select the most likely investigation from the list of options above. Each option may be used once, more than once, or not at all.

❑ **1.** A 70-year-old man is admitted with severe central and epigastric pain and vomiting. On examination he has bruising on his flanks.

❑ **2.** An 18-year-old man has a 2-year history of central abdominal pain, which now has moved to the right iliac fossa. He has had two episodes of loose stools over the past 6 months.

❑ **3.** A middle-aged woman presents with epigastric pain. She has shallow breathing, tachycardia, but is normotensive. She has rheumatoid arthritis and receives regular gold injections and takes oral steroids and diclofenac. She has taken an increased steroid dose over the past week because of a chest infection.

❑ **4.** An elderly woman presents with a history of copious rectal bleeding over a 7-hour period. She is tachycardic and hypotensive.

4.48 Long-term effects of gastrectomy include

❑ A low serum iron
❑ B renal calculi
❑ C osteomalacia
❑ D vitamin B_{12} deficiency
❑ E vitamin C deficiency

4.49 Full-thickness rectal prolapse

- ❑ A has an equal sex incidence
- ❑ B tends to occur at the extremes of life
- ❑ C usually starts as an internal intussusception
- ❑ D may be treated by direct suturing to the sacrum
- ❑ E may cause faecal incontinence

4.50 Carcinoid tumours

- ❑ A may be found incidentally
- ❑ B most commonly occur in the large bowel
- ❑ C are neuroendocrine in origin
- ❑ D secrete bradykinin
- ❑ E may be treated with chemoembolisation

4.51 Hepatic metastases from colorectal cancer

- ❑ A are potentially curable in 25% of cases
- ❑ B best surgical results are achieved by resection along hepatic segmental lines
- ❑ C are not curable using current chemotherapy regimens
- ❑ D are present in about 10% of patients at the time of diagnosis of the primary tumour
- ❑ E are radiosensitive

4.52 Colorectal cancer

- ❑ A is inherited in approximately 40% of cases
- ❑ B is metachronous in 10% of cases
- ❑ C is synchronous in 5% of cases
- ❑ D inevitably occurs in cases of untreated familial adenomatous polypitis (FAP)
- ❑ E clinical stage of disease is the most important prognostic factor

4.53 Barium enema examination of the colon

- ❑ A is as sensitive as colonoscopy for the assessment of polyps
- ❑ B is more sensitive than colonoscopy for the assessment of diverticular disease
- ❑ C can exclude collagenous colitis
- ❑ D single-contrast studies are superior to double-contrast studies in the detection of mucosal abnormalities
- ❑ E is accurate for the assessment of appendiceal pathology

4.54 Theme: Acid–base balance

	pH	PaCO2	HCO3–
A	7.20	3.1	11
B	7.42	6.1	35
C	7.56	3.0	30

For each of the patients described below, select the most likely set of blood gas measurements from the list of options above. Each option may be used once, more than once, or not at all.

❑ **1.** A 68-year-old woman with a history of abdominal pain with rebound tenderness and guarding for 72 hours. She exhibits signs of peritonitis and a WBC of 23 x 10^9/l.

❑ **2.** A 45-year-old woman who had a total abdominal hysterectomy for fibroids is now complaining of shortness of breath 7 days after surgery. There is no history of haemoptysis or pleuritic chest pain.

❑ **3.** A 75-year-old man had an uneventful abdominal aortic aneurysm (AAA) repair 10 days ago. He is known to smoke 30 cigarettes per day.

4.55 Pancreatic carcinoma

❑ A rarely develops before the fifth decade
❑ B is more common in men
❑ C is associated with smoking
❑ D responds well to 5-fluorouracil (5-FU) treatment
❑ E frequently presents with a palpable gallbladder

4.56 The appendix normally

❑ A arises from the posteromedial aspect of the caecum
❑ B lies medial to the right ureter
❑ C has taeniae coli
❑ D lies on the right gonadal vessels
❑ E has an avascular mesoappendix which allows safe dissection

4.57 Insulin

- ❑ A inhibits gluconeogenesis
- ❑ B increases protein synthesis
- ❑ C inhibits potassium entry into cells
- ❑ D is synthesised by C cells of the pancreas
- ❑ E increases glucose uptake by the brain

4.58 Radiological features of Crohn's disease on a barium follow-through include

- ❑ A thinning of the valvulae conniventes
- ❑ B fistulas to other intraperitoneal viscera
- ❑ C rose-thorn ulcers
- ❑ D intramural cysts
- ❑ E thinning of the bowel wall

4.59 The normal function of the colon is in the absorption of

- ❑ A water
- ❑ B sodium
- ❑ C chloride
- ❑ D bicarbonate
- ❑ E bile salts

4.60 In colonic diverticular disease

- ❑ A Asians have an increased incidence of left-sided disease
- ❑ B the diverticula are typically antimesenteric
- ❑ C the diverticula are true rather than pulsion types
- ❑ D the circular muscle of the affected bowel is thickened
- ❑ E the affected bowel is usually elongated

4.61 Theme: Acid–base balance

A Metabolic acidosis
B Metabolic alkalosis
C Normal pH
D Respiratory acidosis
E Respiratory alkalosis

For each of the patients described below, select the most likely acid–base status from the list of options above. Each option may be used once, more than once, or not at all.

❑ **1.** A 70-year-old man with chronic obstructive pulmonary disease collapses on the ward after being admitted with an infective exacerbation.

❑ **2.** A 65-year-old man admitted with epigastric pain, vomiting and jaundice. A serum amylase level of 2000 IU was recorded.

❑ **3.** A 41-year-old woman with shortness of breath and haemoptysis, complaining of chest pain was noted to have unilateral leg swelling 4–6 months after a right upper lobectomy for carcinoma of the lung.

4.62 Resection of the terminal ileum is associated with malabsorption of

❑ A calcium
❑ B vitamin B_{12}
❑ C folic acid
❑ D cholesterol
❑ E bile salts

4.63 The following may be seen in the blood film of a postsplenectomy patient:

❑ A target cells
❑ B punctate basophilia
❑ C Howell–Jolly bodies
❑ D sideroblasts
❑ E rouleaux formation

4.64 Squamous-cell carcinoma of the anal canal

- ❑ A may spread to pelvic lymph nodes
- ❑ B is associated with human papillomavirus infection
- ❑ C characteristically presents with faecal incontinence
- ❑ D is relatively radioresistant
- ❑ E is related to increased dietary fat intake

4.65 Pseudomembranous colitis

- ❑ A may follow the use of cefuroxime
- ❑ B is caused by *Clostridium difficile,* which is a normal commensal of the gut
- ❑ C *Clostridium difficile* toxin can be isolated in the stool of over 90% of affected patients
- ❑ D typically produces grey nodules on the mucosal surface
- ❑ E may progress to toxic megacolon
- ❑ F is best treated by oral erythromycin

4.66 Extraintestinal manifestations of inflammatory bowel disease (IBD) include

- ❑ A exophthalmos
- ❑ B abnormalities of liver function tests
- ❑ C primary sclerosing cholangitis
- ❑ D hepatic adenoma
- ❑ E ankylosing spondylitis
- ❑ F urinary calculi formation

4.67 In cases of severe ulcerative colitis

- ❑ A abdominal signs are unaltered by steroids
- ❑ B the ESR is elevated but the CRP level remains normal
- ❑ C sequential plain AXRs are an important means of patient monitoring
- ❑ D any patient with a colonic diameter of >6.5 cm has toxic megacolon
- ❑ E growth retardation may be a feature in children

4.68 Theme: Investigations of the GI tract

A Proctoscopy
B Fully prepared barium enema
C CT scan
D Colonoscopy
E Small bowel follow-through

For each of the patients described below, select the most likely investigation from the list of options above. Each option may be used once, more than once, or not at all.

❑ **1.** A 60-year-old man, had banding of haemorrhoids 8 weeks previously, and continues to pass dark blood and mucus per rectum.

❑ **2.** A 50-year-old woman with psychiatric problems presents with abdominal distension and absolute constipation.

4.69 Perianal abscess

❑ A is rarely found in the intersphincteric space
❑ B may produce a fistula
❑ C obeys Goodsall's rule
❑ D may be drained internally
❑ E may be associated with diabetes mellitus

4.70 Obturator hernia

❑ A is commoner in men
❑ B may present with a lump in the upper inner aspect of the thigh
❑ C commonly causes knee pain
❑ D is most frequently found at laparotomy
❑ E is repaired by direct apposition of the margins of the defect

4.71 Posterior relations of the stomach include the

❑ A right kidney
❑ B head of the pancreas
❑ C left psoas muscle
❑ D left adrenal gland
❑ E left hemidiaphragm

4.72 Relations of the intrathoracic oesophagus include the

- ❑ A trachea
- ❑ B left lobe of the liver
- ❑ C accessory hemiazygos vein
- ❑ D pericardium
- ❑ E right main bronchus
- ❑ F inferior vena cava

4.73 A Kocher's incision

- ❑ A divides the Colles' fascia
- ❑ B divides only the anterior rectus sheath
- ❑ C divides the external oblique muscle
- ❑ D involves the area innervated by T10 nerve root
- ❑ E divides the fascia transversalis muscle
- ❑ F divides the rectus abdominis muscle

4.74 The lienorenal ligament contains the following:

- ❑ A splenic artery
- ❑ B renal artery
- ❑ C tail of the pancreas
- ❑ D portal vein
- ❑ E splenic vein
- ❑ F left adrenal gland

4.75 Acute diverticulitis of the colon

- ❑ A produces bowel wall thickening, which may be seen on CT
- ❑ B may be accurately diagnosed by Gastrografin enema
- ❑ C settles with intravenous antibiotics alone in 50% of cases
- ❑ D may be treated by colectomy and primary anastomosis
- ❑ E when treated medically recurs in 70% cases
- ❑ F is a premalignant disease

4.76 Anal cancer

❑ A usually arises from anal glands
❑ B is associated with a fivefold increased risk with a history of genital warts
❑ C may present with inguinal lymph node involvement in up to 30% cases
❑ D most commonly presents with a lump
❑ E should ideally be examined under anaesthesia

4.77 Acute pseudocysts of the pancreas

❑ A have a cyst wall composed of fibrous and granulation tissue
❑ B may be found in the mediastinum
❑ C are usually found in the lesser sac
❑ D do not occur following trauma
❑ E cause a persistently raised amylase level in 50% cases

4.78 Zollinger–Ellison syndrome

❑ A usually presents at 50 years of age
❑ B should be suspected if a peptic ulcer is refractory to treatment
❑ C patients typically have ulcers in unusual locations
❑ D is frequently caused by a benign granuloma
❑ E is not amenable to medical management
❑ F can be assessed using an octreotide scan

4.79 Carcinoma of the gallbladder

❑ A usually presents with jaundice
❑ B has an association with gallstones
❑ C has an overall 5-year survival rate of 40%
❑ D is usually an adenocarcinoma
❑ E is effectively treated with chemotherapy

4.80 Dumping syndrome

❑ A may follow gastroenterostomy
❑ B may present with epigastric discomfort, sweating and diarrhoea
❑ C may be avoided by pylorus-preserving surgery
❑ D results from hypo-osmolar solutions reaching the small bowel
❑ E is reduced by eating high-carbohydrate meals frequently

4.81 Theme: Pancreatitis

A Cancer of the head of the pancreas
B Acute-on-chronic pancreatitis
C Biliary obstruction
D Acute pancreatitis
E Pancreatic pseudocyst

For each of the patients described below, select the most likely diagnosis from the list of options above. Each option may be used once, more than once, or not at all.

❑ **1.** A 43-year-old man, with a history of alcohol abuse, presents with pain radiating to his back, which is relieved by leaning forward. He has obstructive jaundice and has recent weight loss.

❑ **2.** A 52-year-old man who drinks 14 units/day and is a heavy smoker presents with acute onset of epigastric pain. He has a history of chronic pancreatitis, steatorrhoea and also has a palpable abdominal mass.

❑ **3.** A 40-year-old man with a history of sudden onset abdominal pain and vomiting has an increased serum amylase level. He has no previous history of pancreatitis.

4.82 During digital rectal examination you can feel the

❑ A ischial tuberosity
❑ B rectovesical pouch
❑ C cervix
❑ D seminal vesicles
❑ E ureter

4.83 The epiploic foramen

❑ A has a superior border formed by the caudate lobe of the liver
❑ B has an inferior border formed by the second part of the duodenum
❑ C has the aorta as a posterior border
❑ D has the gastroduodenal artery as a posterior border
❑ E has the portal vein lying anteriorly
❑ F has the IVC lying inferiorly

4.84 Causes of right upper quadrant (RUQ) pain in a 40-year-old woman include

- ❑ A acute cholecystitis
- ❑ B gastritis
- ❑ C ovarian cyst
- ❑ D lobar pneumonia
- ❑ E *Chlamydia trachomatis* infection

4.85 Following splenectomy

- ❑ A portal vessel pressure increases
- ❑ B thrombocytosis may occur
- ❑ C there is an increased susceptibility to pneumococcal infection
- ❑ D blood supply to the stomach may be at risk

4.86 Causes of mechanical large bowel obstruction

- ❑ A irritable bowel syndrome
- ❑ B solitary rectal ulcer
- ❑ C carcinoma of the colon
- ❑ D diverticular disease
- ❑ E metaplastic polyp
- ❑ F Crohn's disease

4.87 Theme: Cholecystectomy

A Lithotripsy
B Elective cholecystectomy
C Emergency cholecystectomy
D Endoscopic retrograde cholangiopancreatography (ERCP)
E Cholestyramine

For each of the patients described below, select the most likely treatment from the list of options above. Each option may be used once, more than once, or not at all.

❑ **1.** A 77-year-old woman presents with abdominal pain and jaundice. Ultrasound reveals stones in the common bile duct. She is unwell and not fit for theatre.

❑ **2.** A young woman presents to the outpatient department with a history of fat intolerance and abdominal pain in the right upper quadrant. An ultrasound scan reveals that she has gallstones. Upper GI endoscopy was normal.

4.88 Theme: Pancreatic tumour

A Zollinger–Ellison syndrome
B Dumping syndrome
C Insulinoma
D Glucagonoma
E VIPoma

For each of the patients described below, select the most likely pancreatic tumour from the list of options above. Each option may be used once, more than once, or not at all.

❑ **1.** A vicar who missed breakfast swore during his sermon, but felt better after a late breakfast.

❑ **2.** A 52-year-old man with hypercalcaemia suffers from recurrent gastric ulcers.

4.89 In the inguinal region

❑ A the pectineal ligament is also known as Astley Cooper's ligament
❑ B the vas deferens is also known as the duct of Santorini
❑ C the inguinal ligament is also known as Poupart's ligament
❑ D the transversalis fascia is also known as Scarpa's fascia
❑ E Cloquet's node lies within the femoral canal
❑ F the femoral canal is also known as Alcock's canal

4.90 The right suprarenal gland

❑ A lies against the bare area of the liver
❑ B extends behind the inferior vena cava
❑ C receives blood from the right inferior phrenic artery
❑ D drains into the right renal vein
❑ E lies on the 9th rib

4.91 Pancreatic secretion

❑ A has pH >8
❑ B contains lipase
❑ C contains enterokinase
❑ D is typically <200 ml/day

4.92 Ulcerative colitis

- ❑ A total colectomy is usually required by 25 years of age
- ❑ B steroids are used to maintain remission
- ❑ C can be treated with derivatives of salicylic acid
- ❑ D may involve the terminal ileum

4.93 The differential diagnosis of a femoral hernia includes

- ❑ A varicocele
- ❑ B psoas abscess
- ❑ C spigelian hernia
- ❑ D Troisier's node
- ❑ E saphena varix

4.94 Triglycerides

- ❑ A stimulate the secretion of pancreatic enzymes
- ❑ B stimulate insulin secretion
- ❑ C digestion by pancreatic lipase only becomes active in the presence of a cofactor
- ❑ D are hydrolysed into free fatty acids and phospholipids
- ❑ E digestion commences with lipase secretion at the base of the tongue.

4.95 Theme: Side-effects of treatment for inflammatory bowel disease

A Sulfasalazine
B Corticosteroids
C Methotrexate
D Azathioprine
E Metronidazole

For each of the options listed below, select the most likely associated side-effects from the list of drugs above. Each option may be used once, more than once, or not at all.

- ❑ **1.** Irreversible peripheral neuropathy.
- ❑ **2.** Reversible infertility due to oligospermia.
- ❑ **3.** Osteoporosis.
- ❑ **4.** Cataracts.

❑ **5.** Hepatic fibrosis

❑ **6.** Pneumonitis

4.96 Theme: Surgical investigations

A Gastrografin enema
B Abdominal and pelvic CT scan
C Small bowel follow-through
D ERCP
E Abdominal ultrasound
F Colonoscopy
G Barium enema

For each of the conditions listed below, select the most appropriate investigation from the list above. Each option may be used once, more than once, or not at all.

❑ **1.** A suspected, acutely obstructing large bowel cancer.

❑ **2.** Empyema of the gallbladder.

❑ **3.** Colonic diverticular abscess.

❑ **4.** Terminal ileal Crohn's disease.

❑ **5.** Colonic anastomotic leak on day 4 postoperatively.

4.97 Theme: Surgical investigations

A Gastrografin enema
B Abdominal CT scan
C small bowel follow-through
D Endoscopic retrograde cholangiopancreatography (ERCP)
E Abdominal ultrasound
F Barium enema (double contrast)
G Colonoscopy

For each of the following scenarios, select the most appropriate investigation from the list above. Each option may be used once, more than once, or not at all.

❑ **1.** Psoas abscess.

❑ **2.** small bowel tumour.

❑ **3.** Colovesical fistula.

❑ **4.** Pancreatic necrosis.

4.98 Theme: Abdominal disease

A Crohn's disease
B Diverticular disease
C Ulcerative colitis
D Familial adenomatous polyposis
E Peutz–Jeghers' syndrome

For each of the following conditions below, select the most likely associated disease from the list above. Each option may be used once, more than once, or not at all.

❑ **1.** Intra-abdominal desmoids.

❑ **2.** Ankylosing spondylitis.

❑ **3.** Enteroenteric fistulas.

❑ **4.** Perianal sepsis.

❑ **5.** Pyoderma gangrenosum.

❑ **6.** Colovesical fistula.

4.99 Theme: Hernias

A Epigastric hernia
B Spigelian hernia
C Obturator hernia
D Lumbar hernia
E Gluteal hernia
F Sciatic hernia
G Perineal hernia
H Diaphragmatic hernia

For each site of herniation below, select the most likely hernial type from the list above. Each answer may be used once, more than once, or not at all.

❑ **1.** Triangle of Petit.

❑ **2.** Greater sciatic notch.

❑ **3.** Pelvic floor.

❑ **4.** Linea semilunaris.

4.100 Inguinal hernia

❑ A annual death rate from femoral hernias is higher than inguinal hernia in the UK
❑ B management as a day-case surgical procedure is declining
❑ C is less common than femoral hernia in women
❑ D repair may include orchidectomy
❑ E should only be repaired by a mesh technique

4.101 Suitable surgical repairs for a small non-reducible inguinal hernia in a 32-year-old man include

❑ A rat-tailed truss
❑ B laparoscopic extraperitoneal repair
❑ C Shouldice repair
❑ D Lichtenstein mesh repair
❑ E Bassini repair
❑ F herniotomy

4.102 During inguinal hernia repair, the following structures are encountered:

❑ A Scarpa's fascia
❑ B Colles' fascia
❑ C ilioinguinal nerve
❑ D cremasteric muscle
❑ E superior epigastric vein
❑ F iliohypogastric nerve

4.103 Bile salts

- ❑ A may be released by cholecystokinin
- ❑ B decrease bowel motility
- ❑ C increase fat absorption
- ❑ D undergo enterohepatic circulation
- ❑ E are mainly absorbed in the proximal ileum

4.104 Chronic alcohol abuse may present with

- ❑ A Wernicke's encephalopathy
- ❑ B Korsakoff's syndrome
- ❑ C cerebellar ataxia
- ❑ D impotence
- ❑ E Sydenham's chorea
- ❑ F lymphopenia
- ❑ G macrocytosis
- ❑ H menorrhagia

4.105 Features more likely to be associated with Crohn's disease than ulcerative colitis include

- ❑ A stricture formation
- ❑ B obstruction
- ❑ C fistula formation
- ❑ D cancer
- ❑ E perianal involvement

4.106 Crohn's disease is associated with

- ❑ A terminal ileum involvement in over 90% cases
- ❑ B erythema multiforme
- ❑ C skip lesions
- ❑ D cobblestone appearance on contrast enema
- ❑ E uveitis

4.107 Haematoma of the rectus sheath

- ❑ A may occur after a seat-belt injury
- ❑ B may only be diagnosed by a laparotomy
- ❑ C can mimic the signs of diverticulitis
- ❑ D can occur spontaneously
- ❑ E has a high incidence in young, fit men

4.108 Theme: Polyps

A Tubular adenomatous polyps
B Villous adenomatous polyps
C Peutz–Jeghers' polyps
D Metaplastic polyps
E Inflammatory polyps

For each of the descriptions below, select the most appropriate polyp from the list above. Each option may be used once, more than once, or not at all.

❑ **1.** Are usually a consequence of a severe episode of ulcerative colitis.

❑ **2.** Are hamartomas.

❑ **3.** May cause hypokalaemia.

❑ **4.** Have the greatest malignant potential of all colonic polyps.

❑ **5.** Are the commonest type of polyp seen in familial adenomatous polyposis.

4.109 Theme: Gastrointestinal haemorrhage

A Colonoscopy
B Oesophagogastroduodenoscopy
C Selective mesenteric angiography
D Red cell scan
E Double-contrast barium enema
F Single-contrast enema (Gastrografin)
G Laparoscopy
H CT colonography

For each of the patients described below, select the most appropriate investigation from the list above. Each option may be used once, more than once, or not at all.

❑ **1.** A 45-year-old man is admitted to A&E with passage of large clots of fresh blood per rectum. There is no evidence of melaena. He is hypotensive, with a blood pressure of 85/40 mmHg and a pulse rate of 140/min. There is no history of haematemesis but he is a smoker and drinks 20 units of alcohol per week.

❑ **2.** An 85-year-old man is admitted with passage of dark clots per rectum. His blood pressure is 110/70 mmHg and his pulse rate is 90/min. He has recently been complaining of left-sided abdominal pain and a change in bowel habit.

❑ **3.** A 25-year-old man attends the Outpatient Department with three episodes of bright-red rectal bleeding. Rigid sigmoidoscopy and proctoscopy failed to reveal any local causes for the bleeding.

4.110 Theme: Hernias

A Richter's hernia
B Littre's hernia
C Maydl's hernia
D Sliding hernia
E Pantaloon hernia

For each description listed below, select the most appropriate hernia from the list above. Each option may be used once, more than once, or not at all.

❑ **1.** Dual sacs straddling the inferior epigastric vessels.

❑ **2.** Two separate loops of bowel.

❑ **3.** The posterior wall of the hernial sac is formed by a herniating viscus.

❑ **4.** Portion of circumference of the bowel.

❑ **5.** Meckel's diverticulum.

4.111 Faecal incontinence may be seen in patients

❑ A with faecal impaction
❑ B with Cushing's syndrome
❑ C following pelvic radiotherapy for cervical carcinoma
❑ D following parturition
❑ E with anal fistula
❑ F ulcerative colitis

4.112 Theme: Jaundice

A Duodenal carcinoma
B Biliary colic
C Hepatitis C
D Acute cholangitis
E Hepatocellular carcinoma
F Chronic pancreatitis
G Gilbert's disease

For each description listed below, select the most appropriate diagnosis from the list above. Each option may be used once, more than once, or not at all.

❑ **1.** A 30-year-old man, following total colectomy 9 months ago for familial adenomatous polyposis (FAP), now presents with abdominal pain and jaundice; he is passing dark urine and pale stools.

❑ **2.** A 70-year-old man presents with epigastric pain, jaundice, rigors and fever.

❑ **3.** A 40-year-old woman presents with right upper quadrant pain. She is nauseated, but does not have jaundice or rigors.

4.113 Abdominal wound dehiscence

❑ A should be suspected if there is serosanguineous discharge from the wound after 2–3 days
❑ B is more common in midline than paramedian incisions
❑ C affects male patients more commonly than female
❑ D is less common after emergency surgical procedures
❑ E is reduced by separate closure of the peritoneum

4.114 Oesophageal cancer

❑ A is decreasing in incidence
❑ B may be palliated with Nd–YAG laser therapy
❑ C arising in Barrett's oesophagus is usually squamous-cell carcinoma
❑ D is associated with an overall 5-year survival of 10%
❑ E can be accurately staged with endoluminal ultrasonography

4.115 Volvulus of the sigmoid colon

- ❑ A usually occurs in a clockwise direction
- ❑ B is usually diagnosed on a plain abdominal radiograph
- ❑ C is initially treated by reduction with a rigid sigmoidoscope
- ❑ D when associated with gangrene of the sigmoid colon, may be treated by a Hartmann's procedure
- ❑ E has a recurrence rate of 90% with non-operative management

4.116 Colon carcinoma

- ❑ A incidence is increased in Gardner's syndrome
- ❑ B is frequently associated with the human papillomavirus (HPV)
- ❑ C is radioresistant
- ❑ D is best predicted by the size of the tumour
- ❑ E arising in the caecum, tends to present at an earlier stage than in the sigmoid colon

4.117 Theme: Jaundice

A Cholangiocarcinoma
B Gallbladder calculi
C Common bile-duct stone
D Mucocele of the gallbladder
E Empyema of the gallbladder

For each of the patients described below, select the most likely diagnosis from the list of options above. Each option may be used once, more than once, or not at all.

❑ **1.** A 34-year-old woman presents with a palpable right upper quadrant mass. She has a fever and is generally unwell.

❑ **2.** A 30-year-old woman who had an open cholecystectomy presents with obstructive jaundice 48 hours after surgery.

❑ **3.** A 38-year-old obese woman presents with right upper quadrant pain. Ultrasound scanning shows a stone in Hartmann's pouch.

4.118 Rectal carcinoma

❑ A Dukes A is confined to the muscularis propria with no lymph node involvement
❑ B may be treated with preoperative radiotherapy
❑ C mostly originates from ulcers
❑ D usually spreads to inguinal lymph nodes
❑ E may respond to 5-fluorouracil chemotherapy

4.119 Diazepam

❑ A antagonises GABA receptors
❑ B is reversed by naloxone
❑ C causes amnesia
❑ D is broken down to active metabolites
❑ E has a longer half-life than midazolam

4.120 Theme: Pancreatic tumours

A Zollinger–Ellison syndrome
B Glucagonoma
C Insulinoma
D Adenocarcinoma
E Non-secreting, islet-cell tumour

For each of the patients described below, select the most likely diagnosis from the list of options above. Each option may be used once, more than once, or not at all.

❑ **1.** A patient with glossitis and stomatitis has diabetes and a rash on his buttocks.

❑ **2.** A patient 4 weeks after parathyroidectomy presents with loss of consciousness and dizziness.

4.121 The intramural pH of the stomach

❑ A is calculated from the Henderson–Hasselbalch equation
❑ B is considered normal if pH = 7.2
❑ C is dependent on the luminal bicarbonate concentration being equivalent to the plasma bicarbonate concentration
❑ D is increased in a state of metabolic acidosis
❑ E is decreased in profound hypovolaemia

4.122 In the surgical anatomy of the liver

- ❑ A segment I lies to the left of the portal vein
- ❑ B segment II lies medial to the porta hepatis
- ❑ C the caudate lobe lies anterior to the portal vein
- ❑ D the portal vein runs in the anterior border of Winslow's foramen
- ❑ E three hepatic veins divide the liver into four sectors

4.123 Ileoanal pouch

- ❑ A should be offered to all patients who have had a panproctocolectomy
- ❑ B formation should be ideally covered by a defunctioning colostomy
- ❑ C is unlikely to be complicated by an enterocutaneous fistula
- ❑ D is commonly performed following total colectomy for Crohn's disease
- ❑ E produces approximately 6 defecations per 24 hours

4.124 Anal fissure

- ❑ A classically causes predefecatory pain
- ❑ B is found most commonly in women in the sixth decade
- ❑ C is usually anterior in men
- ❑ D may be treated by glyceryl trinitrate cream
- ❑ E is strongly associated with ulcerative colitis
- ❑ F is associated with colorectal carcinoma

4.125 Theme: Jaundice

A Prehepatic jaundice
B Hepatic jaundice
C Posthepatic jaundice

For each of the clinical findings given below, select the correct type of jaundice from the list above. Each option may be used once, more than once, or not at all.

❑ **1.** Bilirubin in the urine.

❑ **2.** History of recent foreign travel.

❑ **3.** Positive Courvoisier's sign.

❑ **4.** Associated pancreatitis.

4.126 The anal canal

- ❑ A lies below the levator ani muscle
- ❑ B has a longitudinal muscular coat
- ❑ C has a lymphatic drainage via the inguinal lymph nodes
- ❑ D has an external sphincter innervated by the pudendal nerve
- ❑ E possesses valves
- ❑ F the anococcygeal body lies anterior

4.127 The mesentery of the small bowel

- ❑ A contains veins which drain directly into the IVC
- ❑ B has a root overlying the left sacroiliac joint
- ❑ C contains autonomic fibres of the vagus nerve
- ❑ D contains arteries that supply the large bowel
- ❑ E overlies the transverse mesocolon

4.128 Theme: Rectal bleeding

A Crohn's disease
B Solitary juvenile polyp
C Familial adenomatous polyposis
D Necrotising enterocolitis
E Intussusception
F Fissure in ano
G Meckel's diverticulum
H Mid-gut volvulus

For each of the clinical scenarios below, select the most likely cause of rectal bleeding from the list above. Each option may be used once, more than once, or not at all.

❑ **1.** A 7-year-old girl presents with weight loss and anaemia.

❑ **2.** A 13-year-old boy presents with lower abdominal pain and shock.

❑ **3.** A 3-year-old boy presents with painless bleeding, mixed with stool.

❑ **4.** A 16-year-old girl presents with painless bleeding, mixed with stool; her father died of colorectal cancer at the age of 35 years.

❑ **5.** A 10-month-old girl with a previous history of intermittent bile-stained vomiting has collapsed.

4.129 Pancreatitis

- ❑ A may cause disseminated intravascular coagulation (DIC)
- ❑ B is usually complicated by pseudocyst formation
- ❑ C may be complicated by hypercalcaemia
- ❑ D may be related to pancreatic divisum
- ❑ E is characterised by back pain relieved by sitting forward

4.130 Theme: Abdominal pain

A Renal adenocarcinoma
B Ureteric colic
C Pelviureteric obstruction
D Leaking abdominal aortic aneurysm

For each of the statements below, select the most likely diagnosis from the list above. Each option may be used once, more than once, or not at all.

❑ **1.** A 45-year-old presents with haematuria, loin pain and a loin mass.

❑ **2.** A 22-year-old experiences loin pain mainly in the morning after drinking four cups of coffee.

❑ **3.** A 70-year-old presents with loin pain, has a pulse rate of 120/min and a BP of 80/60 mmHg.

4.131 The spleen

- ❑ A is related to the left costodiaphragmatic recess
- ❑ B is in contact with the pancreas
- ❑ C must triple in size to be palpable
- ❑ D is attached to the stomach by the lienorenal ligament
- ❑ E the lesser sac extends into its hilum

4.132 In the femoral region the

- ❑ A femoral sheath contains the femoral vessels
- ❑ B femoral canal lies lateral to the femoral vein
- ❑ C femoral canal contains Cloquet's lymph node
- ❑ D femoral ring is the abdominal end of the femoral canal
- ❑ E pubic branch of the inferior epigastric vein replaces the obturator vein in 30% of cases

CHAPTER 5: URINARY SYSTEM AND RENAL TRANSPLANTATION

5.1 The deep perineal pouch in the male contains the

- ❑ A membranous urethra
- ❑ B seminal vesicles
- ❑ C prostatic urethra
- ❑ D sphincter urethra
- ❑ E bulb of the penis
- ❑ F bulbourethral glands
- ❑ G middle rectal artery

5.2 Theme: Loin pain

A Urinary calculi
B Pyelonephritis
C Aortic aneurysm
D Pancreatitis
E Urinary bladder obstruction
F Pelvi-ureteric junction (PUJ) obstruction
G Renal-cell carcinoma

For each of the patients described below, select the most likely diagnosis from the list of options above. Each option may be used once, more than once, or not at all.

❑ **1.** A 30-year-old man presents with loin pain, pyrexia and tachycardia.

❑ **2.** An 18-year-old man presents with pain in his right iliac fossa and microscopic haematuria.

❑ **3.** A woman known to have a previous history of bilateral reflux presents with dysuria, fever and feeling generally unwell.

5.3 In the inguinal region

- ❑ A the inguinal ligament is formed by the in-rolled edge of the internal oblique aponeurosis
- ❑ B the inguinal ligament runs from the anterior inferior iliac spine to the pubic symphysis
- ❑ C the inguinal canal contains a nerve arising from the second and third sacral nerves.
- ❑ D the inferior epigastric artery runs laterally to the deep inguinal ring
- ❑ E a direct inguinal hernia arises medial to the deep inguinal ring

5.4 The external inguinal ring in the male

- ❑ A is formed by a V-shaped slit in the internal oblique aponeurosis
- ❑ B transmits the testicular artery
- ❑ C transmits the cremasteric artery
- ❑ D transmits the femoral branch of the genitofemoral nerve
- ❑ E transmits the pampiniform plexus
- ❑ F transmits the iliohypogastric nerve
- ❑ G transmits the cremasteric muscle

5.5 Horseshoe kidney

- ❑ A is more common in women
- ❑ B usually has a standard blood supply
- ❑ C is more prone to infection
- ❑ D is more prone to trauma
- ❑ E may complicate aortic aneurysm repair

5.6 Theme: Scrotal swellings

A Hydrocele
B Encysted hydrocele of cord
C Varicocele
D Torsion of hydatid of Morgagni
E Epididymo-orchitis
F Inguinoscrotal hernia
G Testicular tumour

For each of the patients described below, select the most likely diagnosis from the list of options above. Each option may be used once, more than once, or not at all.

❑ **1.** A 42-year-old man presents with a left-sided scrotal swelling. You are unable to get above the swelling, it is compressible, increases on standing, but does not have a positive cough impulse.

❑ **2.** An 18-year-old man presents with a sudden onset of testicular pain. On examination you note a firm irregular testis at the apex of the scrotum.

❑ **3.** A 22-year-old patient presents with a scrotal swelling that you are unable to get above, is compressible, increases on standing and has a cough impulse present.

❑ **4.** A patient presents with a painless long-standing scrotal swelling which transilluminates. The swelling is not separate from the testis.

5.7 Acute epididymitis

❑ A is rare before puberty
❑ B has no identifying underlying cause in 50% of cases
❑ C rarely causes a secondary hydrocele
❑ D with urethral discharge is most commonly due to *Chlamydia* spp.
❑ E may lead to testicular atrophy

5.8 Bladder calculi

❑ A usually arise from calculi passed down the ureter
❑ B occur in bladder diverticulae
❑ C classically present with lower abdominal pain
❑ D are commonly associated with UTI
❑ E may lead to transitional-cell carcinoma in long-standing cases

5.9 Prostatic carcinoma

❑ A is the commonest male genitourinary tract malignancy
❑ B has a constant incidence in patients over the age of 65 years
❑ C presents with metastatic disease in over 50% of cases
❑ D androgen antagonists give symptomatic relief in disseminated carcinoma in only 30% of patients
❑ E is usually radiosensitive
❑ F surgical castration reduces circulating androgen levels by about 25%

5.10 Theme: Renal tract calculi

A Extracorporeal shock wave lithotripsy (ESWL)
B Percutaneous nephrostomy
C Nephrectomy
D Percutaneous nephrolithotomy (PCNL)
E Ureteroscopy
F Conservative management

For each of the patients below, select the most appropriate treatment from the list above. Each option may be used once, more than once, or not at all.

❑ **1.** A 24-year-old woman presents with intermittent right loin pain. A mid-stream urine specimen (MSU) confirms microscopic haematuria. A plain radiograph shows a 1.2-cm calculus in the region of the right kidney. An intravenous urogram (IVU) confirms that it lies within the renal pelvis but is not causing obstruction.

❑ **2.** A 45-year-old woman presents with a history of recurrent urinary tract infections (UTIs) and chronic left loin pain. An ultrasound shows a large echogenic mass in the left pelvicalyceal system. A plain kidney and upper bladder (KUB) demonstrates a staghorn calculus. A DMSA scan shows differential split function left:right, 9:91.

❑ **3.** A 31-year-old man presents with colicky left loin pain. He is tachycardic, flushed and has a temperature of 38.5 °C. An intravenous urogram (IVU) shows a 3-mm calculus in the mid-ureter.

5.11 The following are complications of transurethral resection of the prostate (TURP):

❑ A hypernatraemia
❑ B hypothermia
❑ C secondary haemorrhage
❑ D incontinence
❑ E increased risk of stroke

5.12 Renal calculi

- ❑ A usually present in the fourth decade of life
- ❑ B are usually due to hyperparathyroidism
- ❑ C may be caused by *Enterobacteria* spp.
- ❑ D in the renal pelvis may be treated with ESWL
- ❑ E produce microscopic haematuria in 50% cases

5.13 Theme: Benign prostatic hyperplasia

A Doxazosin
B Prazosin
C TURP
D Urethral catheterization
E Retropubic (open) prostatectomy
F Radical prostatectomy
G Trial without catheter

For each of the patients below, select the most appropriate treatment from the list above. Each option may be used once, more than once, or not at all.

❑ **1.** A 71-year-old man presents with acute urinary retention. Upon catheterisation his residual volume was 800 ml. His creatinine concentration on admission was 350 mmol/l. Following management of a postobstructive diuresis the creatinine concentration returned to 90 mmol/l. Digital rectal examination suggests a large benign prostate. A transrectal ultrasound shows a prostate volume of 180 ml with no hypoechoic areas.

❑ **2.** A 56-year-old man presents with moderate lower urinary tract symptoms. He has persistent macroscopic haematuria. A digital rectal examination shows a large benign-feeling prostate. MSU, cytology, an IVU and flexible cystoscopy were negative for transitional-cell carcinoma. He wishes to have another child in the near future.

❑ **3.** A 59-year-old man presents with vague abdominal pain. An ultrasound showed bilateral hydronephrosis with a postmicturition residual volume of 1500 ml. His serum creatinine was normal.

5.14 The male urethra

- ❑ A has a prostatic part bounded by the internal and external urethral sphincter
- ❑ B has a spongy part which, when ruptured, leaks urine over the abdomen subcutaneously
- ❑ C has a 90° angle in its membranous part
- ❑ D is narrowest at the external urethral meatus
- ❑ E has a penile part invested by the erectile tissue of the corpora cavernosa

5.15 Neuropathic bladder dysfunction is associated with

- ❑ A spina bifida
- ❑ B diabetes mellitus
- ❑ C abdominal hysterectomy
- ❑ D anterior resection
- ❑ E vesicoureteric reflux

5.16 Theme: Testicular tumours

A Close follow-up
B Testicular biopsy
C Antiandrogen therapy
D Radiotherapy
E Chemotherapy
F Radical orchidectomy
G Retroperitoneal lymph node dissection

For each of the patients below, select the most appropriate subsequent treatment from the list above. Each option may be used once, more than once, or not at all.

❑ **1.** A 34-year-old man presents with a hard, irregular swelling of his right testis. Alpha-fetoprotein and β-hCG are normal. An ultrasound shows a heterogenous mass in the upper pole of the right testis. Investigations reveal no lymphadenopathy. A radical orchidectomy confirms a testicular seminoma which is completely excised.

❑ **2.** A 22-year-old man presents with a hard, irregular swelling of his right testis. Ultrasound suggests a right testicular tumour and a left testis containing hypoechoic areas and microcalcification. A right radical orchidectomy and a left testicular biopsy are performed. Histology shows the right testicular seminoma is completely excised. A widespread, low-grade, intratubular, germ-cell neoplasia is found on the left.

❑ **3.** A 24-year-old man underwent an orchidectomy for a non-seminatous, germ-cell tumour. A postoperative CT scan shows a 7-cm mass of retroperitoneal lymphadenopathy. After a course of chemotherapy his tumour markers normalise and CT scanning shows shrinkage of the nodal mass to 3.5 cm.

5.17 Carcinoma of the prostate

❑ A is the commonest adult male tumour in the UK
❑ B occurs in >30% of men over 50 years of age
❑ C 70% of tumours arise in the peripheral zone
❑ D is more common in white men
❑ E has a threefold increased risk if two first-degree relatives are affected

5.18 Urinary incontinence

❑ A may be secondary to urinary retention
❑ B following TURP almost always implies iatrogenic damage to the external urinary sphincter
❑ C in woman may be treated with a Prolene tape slung around the mid-urethra
❑ D complete incontinence is seen in approximately 3% of cases following radical prostatectomy
❑ E can be treated by pelvic floor exercises if due to stress incontinence

5.19 Theme: Transitional-cell carcinoma

A transurethral resection (TURBT)
B Intravesical mitomycin
C Intravesical BCG
D M-VAC chemotherapy
E Radical cystectomy
F Nephrectomy
G Nephroureterectomy
H Cystoscopy

For each of the patients below, select the most appropriate treatment from the list above. Each option may be used once, more than once, or not at all.

❏ **1.** A 64-year-old man presents with haematuria. An IVU shows normal upper tracts with a filling defect in the bladder. Flexible cystoscopy confirms a tumour.

❏ **2.** A 58-year-old woman with a history of superficial bladder cancer is found to have an irregular filling defect in the right renal pelvis. CT confirms a solid mass.

❏ **3.** A fit 55-year-old man presents with haematuria. Investigations reveal a bladder tumour. A TURBT shows a muscle-invasive bladder cancer (stage T_2) and EUA confirms the bladder is mobile. CT scanning shows three 2–3-cm pelvic lymph nodes.

5.20 The following stones form in acidic urine:

❏ A cysteine
❏ B staghorn calculi
❏ C urate calculi
❏ D calcium phosphate
❏ E struvite calculi

5.21 Theme: Imaging

A Plain KUB
B IVU
C Ultrasound
D Cystogram
E Retrograde ureterogram
F DMSA scan
G DTPA scan
H Spiral CT scan

For each of the patients below, select the most appropriate treatment from the list above. Each option may be used once, more than once, or not at all.

❑ **1.** A 34-year-old obese man presents with a sudden onset of colicky right loin pain radiating to his groin. He has microscopic haematuria. He has a history of severe anaphylaxis with intravenous contrast. An ultrasound scan is unhelpful due to his obesity.

❑ **2.** A 45-year-old woman has a right staghorn calculus on plain KUB. An IVU shows this kidney fails to excrete contrast. An ultrasound scan shows the kidney has a thin parenchyma without evidence of hydronephrosis.

❑ **3.** A 22-year-old woman presents with a history of left loin pain shortly after drinking alcohol. An ultrasound scan shows hydronephrosis with a normal calibre ureter. An IVU shows a narrowing at the pelviureteric junction.

5.22 Pelvi-ureteric junction (PUJ) obstruction

❑ A is more common in boys
❑ B is more common on the right
❑ C is best detected with a DMSA scan
❑ D when detected antenatally does not usually require in-utero treatment

5.23 Concerning treatment of organ-confined prostate cancer

- ❑ A if treated conservatively has an 85% disease-specific survival at 10 years
- ❑ B radical prostatectomy is associated with a 15% complete incontinence rate
- ❑ C radical prostatectomy may be performed through a perineal or retropubic approach
- ❑ D cryotherapy is a widely accepted treatment option
- ❑ E brachytherapy is the implantation of radioactive seeds within the prostate

5.24 Theme: Renal transplant

A Acute rejection
B Hyperacute rejection
C Chronic rejection
D Blood group mismatch

Match the following concerning transplantation. Each option may be used once, more than once, or not at all.

❑ **1.** The humoral system is responsible for this.

❑ **2.** Cellular immunity is responsible for this.

❑ **3.** This causes haemolysis.

❑ **4.** Presensitisation is responsible for this.

5.25 The prostate gland

- ❑ A is transversed by ejaculatory ducts
- ❑ B is lateral to levator ani
- ❑ C receives a blood supply from the pudendal artery
- ❑ D has the ureters lying laterally
- ❑ E has a venous drainage to the internal vertebral plexus
- ❑ F contains the widest part of the urethra

5.26 In the staging of prostate cancer

- ❑ A biopsy may detect stage T_{1c} prostate cancer
- ❑ B seminal vesical involvement is stage T_{3a}
- ❑ C tumour detected following TURP is stage T_{1a} if <15% chips involved
- ❑ D palpable tumour involving both lobes is T_{2b}
- ❑ E extracapsular extension, not involving seminal vesicals, is T_{3b}

PRACTICE PAPER 1 – MULTIPLE CHOICE QUESTIONS

Time allowed: 2½ hrs

1 Osteosarcoma

- ❑ A affects the epiphysis of the long bones
- ❑ B usually presents between the ages of 30 and 50 years
- ❑ C is a recognised complication of Paget's disease
- ❑ D produces increased bone formation
- ❑ E complicates osteochondroma

2 Conduction deafness is caused by

- ❑ A Paget's disease of the bone
- ❑ B an acoustic neuroma
- ❑ C otosclerosis
- ❑ D a fracture through the petrous temporal bone
- ❑ E otitis media

3 The posterior third of the tongue has

- ❑ A filiform papillae
- ❑ B fungiform papillae
- ❑ C lymphoid tissue
- ❑ D a sensory innervation from the internal laryngeal nerve
- ❑ E a sensory innervation from the chordae tympani

4 The ilioinguinal nerve

- ❑ A lies posterior to the kidney
- ❑ B is entirely sensory
- ❑ C passes through the deep inguinal ring
- ❑ D passes through the superficial inguinal ring
- ❑ E supplies sensation to the scrotum
- ❑ F may be damaged by a gridiron incision

5 The colon can

- ❑ A absorb up to 5 litres of water a day
- ❑ B produce short-chain fatty acids from cellulose
- ❑ C go into ileus following a laparotomy
- ❑ D exchange Cl^- and HCO_3^-

6 The rectum

- ❑ A normally drains into the superficial inguinal lymph nodes
- ❑ B has a venous drainage into the superior mesenteric vein
- ❑ C has a peritoneal mesentery
- ❑ D drains to the mesenteric lymph nodes
- ❑ E is supplied by the middle rectal artery

7 Carpal tunnel syndrome

- ❑ A is a recognised complication of rheumatoid arthritis
- ❑ B is frequently caused by a cervical rib
- ❑ C spares the abductor pollicis brevis
- ❑ D should be diagnosed by nerve conduction studies
- ❑ E is treated by division of the extensor retinaculum

8 Meckel's diverticulum

- ❑ A is invariably found in the jejunum
- ❑ B is a recognised cause of malabsorption
- ❑ C should not be removed if found incidentally
- ❑ D may present with rectal bleeding
- ❑ E may lead to macrocytic anaemia
- ❑ F is found in over 20% of the general population
- ❑ G is a true diverticulum
- ❑ H is associated with a patent urachus

9 The kidney is in direct contact with the

- ❑ A costodiaphragmatic angle of the pleural cavity
- ❑ B subcostal nerve
- ❑ C psoas muscle
- ❑ D ilioinguinal nerve
- ❑ E cisterna chyli

10 Enterovesical fistulas

- ❑ A are secondary to diverticular disease in approximately 50% of cases
- ❑ B present with pneumaturia in over 50% of cases
- ❑ C lead to faecaluria in 75% of cases
- ❑ D are secondary to colorectal cancer in approximately 50% of cases
- ❑ E rarely complicate Crohn's disease

11 Amyloidosis is seen in

- ❑ A papillary carcinoma of thyroid
- ❑ B acute pancreatitis
- ❑ C multiple myeloma
- ❑ D dialysis patients
- ❑ E rheumatoid arthritis

12 The femoral artery

- ❑ A is anterior to the vein in the adductor canal
- ❑ B has no branch in the adductor canal
- ❑ C is posterior to the psoas muscle
- ❑ D is posterior to the adductor brevis
- ❑ E is posterior to the adductor longus
- ❑ F passes through the adductor longus
- ❑ G is posterior to the femoral vein in the upper thigh

13 The tibial nerve

- ❑ A gives off the sural nerve
- ❑ B lies superficial to the artery in the popliteal fossa
- ❑ C lies lateral to the popliteal artery throughout its course
- ❑ D if damaged will result in loss of dorsiflexion of the foot
- ❑ E supplies the knee joint

14 Recognised complications of acute tonsillitis include

- ❑ A cholesteatoma
- ❑ B acute glomerulonephritis
- ❑ C quinsy
- ❑ D endotoxaemia
- ❑ E vocal cord palsy

15 ECG changes in pulmonary embolism include

- ❑ A left bundle-branch block
- ❑ B left axis deviation
- ❑ C T-wave inversion in V1–3
- ❑ D R wave V6
- ❑ E atrial fibrillation prolonged S wave V1

16 Epigastric hernia

- ❑ A is most common in children
- ❑ B affects men 3 times more frequently than women
- ❑ C is rarely multiple
- ❑ D usually contains omentum
- ❑ E normally requires repair with Prolene mesh

17 The linea semilunaris of the rectus sheath

- ❑ A is crossed by the inferior epigastric vessels
- ❑ B has an upper attachment overlying the gallbladder
- ❑ C is one of the preferred lines of incision in abdominal surgery
- ❑ D is formed by interdigitation of the internal and external oblique aponeuroses
- ❑ E is crossed by the medial umbilical ligament
- ❑ F can be involved in a spigelian hernia
- ❑ G forms one side of Hesselbach's triangle

18 Cystic fibrosis

- ❑ A is a cause of intestinal obstruction
- ❑ B is an abnormality of all exocrine glands
- ❑ C is an abnormality of calcium channels
- ❑ D affects 1:5000 live births
- ❑ E patients may require pancreatin supplements

19 Bladder cancer

- ❑ A is most commonly caused worldwide by exposure to chemical carcinogens
- ❑ B muscle-invasive bladder cancer is associated with abnormalities of chromosome 17
- ❑ C carcinoma in situ has a better prognosis than superficial papillary tumours (G1pTa)
- ❑ D treatment of most bladder tumours is by cystectomy
- ❑ E orthoptic bladder reconstruction is contraindicated in patients with impaired renal function

20 The scalp region

- ❑ A is exclusively supplied from branches of the external carotid artery
- ❑ B contains the C1 dermatome
- ❑ C is tightly attached to the cranium
- ❑ D contains lymph nodes
- ❑ E has a motor innervation from the facial nerve

21 Extraintestinal manifestations of Gardner's syndrome include

- ❑ A osteomas
- ❑ B erythema marginatum
- ❑ C multinodular goitre
- ❑ D epidermoid cysts
- ❑ E tenosynovitis

22 The third part of the duodenum lies

- ❑ A posterior to the superior mesenteric vessels
- ❑ B immediately anterior to the right renal artery
- ❑ C posterior to the root of the mesentery of the small bowel
- ❑ D anterior to the right ureter
- ❑ E anterior to the inferior mesenteric artery

23 Dupuytren's contracture

- ❑ A is associated with alcoholism
- ❑ B is a contracture of the flexor tendons of the hand
- ❑ C most frequently involves the fingers on the ulnar side of the hand
- ❑ D is more common in females
- ❑ E is associated with phenytoin treatment

24 Maxillary carcinoma can present with

- ❑ A ptosis
- ❑ B Horner's syndrome
- ❑ C epistaxis
- ❑ D proptosis
- ❑ E trismus
- ❑ F diplopia

25 The pancreas

- ❑ A overlies the right kidney
- ❑ B lies in the transpyloric plane
- ❑ C has an uncinate process lying anterior to the superior mesenteric vein
- ❑ D gives attachment to the transverse mesocolon
- ❑ E has the inferior mesenteric vein passing behind the neck

26 A patient presents with numbness in the first, second and third toes. The nerves contributing to the numbness include

- ❑ A the medial plantar nerve
- ❑ B the lateral plantar nerve
- ❑ C the superficial peroneal nerve
- ❑ D the sural nerve

27 The following are features of the postphlebitic syndrome:

- ❑ A cellulitis
- ❑ B groin pain
- ❑ C ulcers on calf
- ❑ D ankle oedema
- ❑ E decreased ankle brachial pressure index

28 Metastatic prostatic cancer

- ❑ A is best treated with chemotherapy
- ❑ B diethylstilbestrol therapy may be effective
- ❑ C strontium may be used to reduce pain from widespread bone metastasis
- ❑ D bicalutamide causes painful gynaecomastia
- ❑ E LHRH analogues may cause distressing hot flushes

29 The nasopharynx

- ❑ A receives a sensory nerve supply from the glossopharyngeal nerve
- ❑ B contains the pharyngeal tonsil
- ❑ C is ridged by the palatopharyngeal fold
- ❑ D has the internal carotid artery lying against its wall
- ❑ E contains the pyramidal fossa
- ❑ F has a communication with the oropharynx that is closed during swallowing

30 In a 10-year-old child with an 11-month history of a midline swelling just below the hyoid bone

- ❑ A a Trucut biopsy is a useful test
- ❑ B the swelling is most likely to be a thyroglossal cyst
- ❑ C an ultrasound scan is the most useful first-line test
- ❑ D a technetium scan is essential
- ❑ E the swelling will resolve spontaneously

31 Compared with the lower end of the ileum, the upper end of the jejunum has

- ❑ A a thicker wall
- ❑ B less fat at the mesenteric border
- ❑ C fewer circular folds
- ❑ D a wider lumen
- ❑ E more aggregated lymphatic follicles (Peyer's patches)
- ❑ F more arterial arcades

32 Intracapsular fractures of the femoral neck

- ❑ A are best treated with a dynamic hip screw if markedly displaced
- ❑ B are best treated with a hemiarthroplasty if markedly displaced
- ❑ C can be treated by closed reduction and the insertion of cannulated screws
- ❑ D may be pathological
- ❑ E most commonly occur through a metastatic deposit

33 Carotid body tumour

- ❑ A biopsy is essential for diagnosis
- ❑ B is investigated by angiography
- ❑ C is a cause of syncope
- ❑ D arise from the vessel wall
- ❑ E is more common in people living at high altitude

34 In oesophageal atresia

- ❑ A the incidence is 1 in 1000
- ❑ B gas is never present in the bowel
- ❑ C primary end-to-end anastomosis can be formed where there is a narrow gap between the oesophageal ends
- ❑ D colonic implantation may be necessary
- ❑ E is rarely associated with a tracheal fistula

35 Absolute indications for TURP include

- ❑ A obstructive uropathy with renal impairment
- ❑ B bladder calculus
- ❑ C recurrent prostatitis
- ❑ D persistent haematuria of prostatic origin
- ❑ E residual volume of >200 ml

36 The spermatic cord contains the

- ❑ A pampiniform plexus
- ❑ B vas deferens
- ❑ C testicular artery
- ❑ D dartos muscles
- ❑ E femoral branch of the genitofemoral nerve
- ❑ F ilioinguinal nerve

37 The medial ligament of the ankle

- ❑ A comprises 3 separate bands
- ❑ B is damaged in a 'sprained' ankle
- ❑ C inserts into the calcaneum
- ❑ D has a superficial part
- ❑ E may be associated with an avulsion fracture on X-ray

38 Postsplenectomy sepsis

- ❑ A is more common in adults than in children
- ❑ B may be due to *Streptococcus pneumoniae*
- ❑ C may be due to *Haemophilus influenzae*
- ❑ D may be prevented by daily penicillin
- ❑ E may be due to *Neisseria meningitidis*

39 Intrascrotal testicular torsion

- ❑ A can be reliably diagnosed by ultrasound
- ❑ B is associated with a poor outcome if the delay is more than 6 hours
- ❑ C orchidopexy of the other testicle is required
- ❑ D once successfully repaired has no added risk of future malignancy

40 The IVC (abdominal)

- ❑ A runs in the free edge of the lesser omentum
- ❑ B ascends to the right of the aorta
- ❑ C may be directly in contact with the right suprarenal gland
- ❑ D forms the posterior wall of the epiploic foramen
- ❑ E receives direct drainage from both the right and left suprarenal veins

41 Concerning renal transplantation

- ❑ A the donor kidney is usually sited in an intraperitoneal position
- ❑ B transplantation of a left donor kidney is more technically demanding
- ❑ C a large postoperative lymphocele is treated with peritoneal windowing
- ❑ D graft survival following living donor transplant is equivalent to that of cadaveric transplants
- ❑ E patients with a history of treated primary brain tumour are suitable donors

42 The processus vaginalis

- ❑ A is formed by visceral peritoneum
- ❑ B forms a sac in which the testis descends through the inguinal canal
- ❑ C when present in adults, predisposes to direct inguinal hernia
- ❑ D forms the tunica vaginalis in the adult
- ❑ E invests the adult vas deferens

43 Dislocation of the shoulder

- ❑ A is associated with damage to the radial nerve
- ❑ B is associated with damage to the axillary nerve
- ❑ C usually requires open reduction
- ❑ D requires a postreduction X-ray
- ❑ E requires 2 views for accurate diagnosis

44 Indications for endoscopic retrograde cholangiopancreatography (ERCP) include

- ❑ A cholelithiasis
- ❑ B pancreatic pseudocyst
- ❑ C empyema of the gallbladder
- ❑ D ascending cholangitis
- ❑ E pancreatic divisum

45 The adductor canal

❑ A is bounded in part by the vastus lateralis
❑ B contains the saphenous nerve
❑ C contains the deep femoral artery
❑ D contains the nerve to the vastus medialis
❑ E contains an artery that forms an anastomosis around the knee joint
❑ F contains the nerve that supplies tensor fascia lata

46 Pleomorphic adenoma of the parotid gland

❑ A is the commonest parotid tumour
❑ B has a true capsule
❑ C is a recognised cause of facial nerve palsy
❑ D is effectively treated with radiotherapy
❑ E does not recur after surgical excision

47 Faecal incontinence may be caused by

❑ A spina bifida
❑ B anal warts
❑ C haemorrhoidectomy
❑ D Cushing's syndrome
❑ E irritable bowel syndrome

48 The typical rib has

❑ A an angle at its anterior end
❑ B a costal groove on its superior border
❑ C a tubercle between the head and neck
❑ D an articulation with two vertebrae
❑ E an angle which is the likeliest part to fracture in thoracic trauma

49 Carcinoma of the gallbladder

❑ A is the most common malignancy of the biliary tract
❑ B is usually diagnosed by ultrasound
❑ C is strongly associated with gallstones
❑ D is associated with gallbladder polyps
❑ E has a good response to adjuvant chemotherapy

50 In the orbit the

- ❑ A supraorbital nerve passes through the superior orbital fissure
- ❑ B ophthalmic artery passes through the superior orbital fissure
- ❑ C optic nerve is surrounded by pia, arachnoid and dura
- ❑ D frontal nerve passes through the tendinous ring
- ❑ E nasociliary nerve supplies the cornea
- ❑ F inferior branch of the oculomotor nerve when damaged causes ptosis

51 Torsion of the testis

- ❑ A can be excluded by colour Doppler ultrasound
- ❑ B when found at exploration, should always have the contralateral testis fixed
- ❑ C is most commonly seen between 8 and 10 years of age
- ❑ D the testis may be viable after 24 hours
- ❑ E is usually extravaginal when occurring in adolescents

52 Axillary artery

- ❑ A has branches in its first part
- ❑ B passes through deep fascia
- ❑ C is a continuation of the subclavian artery
- ❑ D and all its branches are usually encountered in an axillary dissection
- ❑ E commences at the lateral border of the second rib

53 Upper limb injuries in children

- ❑ A supracondylar fractures result in valgus deformity
- ❑ B medial epicondylar avulsion is associated with radial nerve injury
- ❑ C pulled elbow is common at 6 years of age
- ❑ D lateral condyle fracture may produce an ulnar palsy

54 The lesser omentum

- ❑ A is supplied by gastroepiploic arteries
- ❑ B is attached to the liver in the fissure of the ligamentum venosum
- ❑ C encloses the right gastric vessels
- ❑ D has the common hepatic bile duct in its free edge
- ❑ E is attached to the first part of the duodenum
- ❑ F has considerable mobility

55 In Crohn's disease

❑ A smoking confers a degree of protection
❑ B smoking does not alter the risk of postoperative recurrence after surgery
❑ C viruses have been shown to have a definite causal relationship
❑ D 25% of patients have a positive family history
❑ E the risk of a child of an affected patient developing Crohn's disease is approximately 25%

56 Sjögren's syndrome

❑ A is associated with rheumatoid arthritis
❑ B may follow a parotidectomy
❑ C is an autoimmune condition
❑ D causes lymphocyte infiltration in the parotid gland
❑ E causes dry eyes and dry mouth

57 The following are found during an approach to the right subclavian artery:

❑ A stellate ganglion
❑ B vagus nerve
❑ C phrenic nerve
❑ D scalenus anterior
❑ E thoracic duct

58 Acute cholecystitis

❑ A may occur in the absence of gallstones
❑ B is a contraindication to laparoscopic cholecystectomy in the first 48 hours
❑ C typically causes a 'hot spot' on an HIDA scan
❑ D is a recognised cause of peritonitis
❑ E complicated by empyema, can be treated by percutaneous drainage

59 In the female reproductive tract

❑ A the ovarian artery supplies the fallopian tube
❑ B most of the anterior surface of the uterus is covered by peritoneum
❑ C ureteric calculi are palpable per vaginum
❑ D the ovary lies posterior to the broad ligament
❑ E lymph drains from the uterine tubes to the superficial inguinal lymph nodes
❑ F the major arterial supply of the uterus originates from the internal iliac artery
❑ G the suspensory ligament of the ovary is a remnant of the gubernaculum

60 The lower urinary tract

❑ A receives a parasympathetic supply from S2–S4
❑ B is supplied by the obturator nerve
❑ C receives a sympathetic supply via the hypogastric plexus
❑ D is supplied by the perineal branch of the pudendal nerve
❑ E the detrusor muscle is under parasympathetic control

61 An abscess in the temporal lobe may cause

❑ A epilepsy
❑ B visual disturbances
❑ C problems with balance
❑ D problems with speech recognition
❑ E meningitis

62 Compartment syndrome

❑ A is caused by increased pressure within a myofascial compartment
❑ B can be treated expectantly in the first instance
❑ C can be investigated with an intracompartmental pressure monitor
❑ D may be associated with a warm, pink extremity
❑ E does not occur in children

63 The cephalic vein

- ❑ A forms in the area of the anatomical snuffbox
- ❑ B is deep to the cutaneous nerve of the forearm
- ❑ C is medial to the biceps muscle
- ❑ D forms the axillary vein by joining the basilic vein
- ❑ E lies on the ulnar aspect of the wrist
- ❑ F has no valves

64 Ulcerative colitis

- ❑ A only affects the mucosa and submucosa layers of the bowel
- ❑ B usually spares the rectum
- ❑ C is associated with an increased incidence of malignancy
- ❑ D is associated with granulomatous inflammation
- ❑ E rarely causes abdominal pain

65 Extracorporeal shock-wave lithotripsy (ESWL)

- ❑ A is contraindicated in pregnancy
- ❑ B is contraindicated in children
- ❑ C can cause Steinstrasse
- ❑ D piezoceramic machines are safe in patients with pacemakers
- ❑ E pretreatment insertion of a ureteric stent is recommended if the stone bulk is >1.5 cm

PRACTICE PAPER 1 – EXTENDED MATCHING QUESTIONS

Theme: Treatment of thyroid disease

A Carbimazole
B Propylthiouracil
C Radio-iodine
D Thyroxine
E Subtotal thyroidectomy

For each of the patients described below, choose the most suitable treatment from the list of options above. Each option may be used once, more than once, or not at all.

❑ **66** A 50-year-old woman presents with smooth diffuse goitre. She has signs of hyperthyroidism, including thyroid acropachy.

❑ **67** A 28-year-old pregnant woman presents with symptoms and signs of thyrotoxicosis.

❑ **68** An 18-year-old woman, thyrotoxic, for whom antithyroid drugs have failed.

Theme: Shoulder pain

A Supraspinatus tendonitis
B Supraspinatus rupture
C Subacromial bursitis
D Biceps rupture
E Acromioclavicular joint disruptions

For each of the patients described below, choose the most suitable diagnosis from the list of options above. Each option may be used once, more than once, or not at all.

❑ **69** A 52-year-old plasterer complains of a 1-year history of shoulder pain and difficulty in lifting his arm up whilst performing his job. On examination he had marked tenderness over the acromium. He has to bend over to the affected side to initiate shoulder abduction. He has no difficulty in passive abduction of his arm.

❑ **70** A 32-year-old man presents with a 1-month history of shoulder pain especially on lifting the arm. On examination he has marked tenderness lateral to the acromial process with a painful arc of 60–120°.

Theme: Low back pain

- A Prolapsed intervertebral disc
- B Muscle strain
- C Facet joint arthrosis
- D Osteoporotic collapse
- E Metastatic disease
- F Spondylolisthesis
- G Discitis

For each of the clinical situations described below, please select the most likely diagnosis from the list above. Each option may be used once, more than once, or not at all.

❑ **71** A teenage boy presents to his GP with a 6-month history of increasing pain and stiffness in his lower lumbar spine. There is no history of trauma although he is an active sportsman. His lumbar spine is stiff to examination and there is bilateral limitation of straight leg raise with pain in the hamstring muscles.

❑ **72** A young man wakes up one morning complaining of pain in his lower back. The day before he had been redecorating his bedroom. There are no nerve root signs but his back is very stiff.

❑ **73** An active 88-year-old woman has had some back pain since she stumbled over her own doorstep 6 weeks ago. Her back was initially stiff but she feels there has been some improvement over the last 2 weeks.

❑ **74** A 3-year-old baby girl refuses to walk. Her symptoms began last night and she is irritable and unwell. Examination of her lower limbs is entirely normal but percussion of her lumbar spine causes her to cry.

❑ **75** A 45-year-old man gives a 3-month history of low back pain, which has become progressively worse such that he is now in agony and cannot get comfortable. The pain radiates to both buttocks and neurological examination suggests there are problems with the sacral nerve roots.

Theme: Complications of hip surgery

- A Death
- B Pulmonary embolus, no prophylaxis
- C Urinary retention, male
- D DVT, no prophylaxis
- E Wound infection without prophylaxis

Match the postoperative risk with the complication for hip replacement. Each option may be used once, more than once, or not at all.

- ❑ **76** 5–10%
- ❑ **77** <1%
- ❑ **78** 1–5%
- ❑ **79** 60%
- ❑ **80** 10–20%

Theme: Anatomy of the joints in the head and neck

- A Atlanto-occipital
- B Temporomandibular
- C Intervertebral disc
- D Cricothyroid
- E Coronal suture
- F Cricoarytenoid
- G Atlantoaxial

For each of the statements below, select the most likely joint from the list above. Each option may be used once, more than once, or not at all.

- ❑ **81** Movements at this joint lengthen the vocal cords.
- ❑ **82** This is a secondary cartilagenous joint.
- ❑ **83** Subserves a rotatory movement whose axis is outside the joint.
- ❑ **84** Flexion of the head occurs at this joint.

Theme: Paediatric conditions

A Pyloric stenosis
B Replicated bowel
C Meckel's diverticulum
D Intussusception

For each of the patients described below, select the most likely diagnosis from the list of options above. Each option may be used once, more than once, or not at all.

❑ **85** A 2-year-old presents with bilious vomiting, per rectum bleeding and a sausage-shaped mass in the abdomen

❑ **86** A 2-month-old presents with non-bilious projectile vomiting after feeds.

❑ **87** A 5-year-old presents with bilious vomiting and per rectum bleeding.

Theme: Neonatal surgical diagnoses

A Hirschsprung's disease
B Oesophageal atresia
C Tracheo-oesophageal fistula
D Imperforate anus
E Duodenal atresia
F Gastroschisis
G Exomphalos
H Mid-gut volvulus
I Necrotising enterocolitis (NEC)

For each of the clinical scenarios given below, select the most likely diagnosis from the list above. Each option may be used once, more than once, or not at all.

❑ **88** A male infant with trisomy 21, born at term, presents with abdominal distension, bile-stained vomiting and collapse. There has been no passage of meconium.

❑ **89** An antenatal observation of intestine and liver outside the fetal abdomen.

❑ **90** A previously well male infant, 6 weeks old and born at 35 weeks' gestation, presents with bile-stained vomiting.

❑ **91** A 4-hour-old female infant noted to be 'frothy', was born to a mother with polyhydramnios during pregnancy.

❑ **92** An 8-day-old female infant presents with respiratory distress at each oral feed.

Theme: Anatomy of abdominal vasculature

A Inferior mesenteric vein
B Superior mesenteric vein
C Left gastric vein
D Right renal artery
E Left renal vein
F Gastroduodenal artery
G Portal vein
H Left suprarenal artery
I Left colic artery
J Ileocolic artery
K Splenic artery
L Middle colic artery
M Superior mesenteric artery
N Left gonadal vein

For each of the statements below, select the most likely option from the list above. Each option may be used once, more than once, or not at all.

❑ **93** Drains the left suprarenal gland.

❑ **94** Supplies the caecum.

❑ **95** Lies to the left of the superior mesenteric vein.

❑ **96** Supplies the fundus of the stomach.

Theme: Anatomy of the inguinal canal

A Anterior wall
B Roof
C Posterior wall
D Floor

For each of the combinations of structures listed below, select the most appropriate portion of the inguinal canal they form from the list above. Each option may be used once, more than once, or not at all.

❑ **97** Inguinal and lacunar ligaments.

❑ **98** Internal oblique and the aponeurosis of the external oblique.

❑ **99** Medial part of the conjoint tendon and fascia transversalis.

❑ **100** Internal oblique, transversus abdomini muscles and conjoint tendon.

Theme: Infective and non-infective intestinal inflammation

A Amoebic dysentery
B *Yersinia* enterocolitis
C Pseudomembranous colitis
D Infective colitis
E Diversion colitis

For each of the statements below, select the most likely form of intestinal inflammation from the list above. Each option may be used once, more than once, or not at all.

❑ **101** Is associated with an acute ileitis and inflamed mesenteric lymph nodes.

❑ **102** The main histological features are oedema of the lamina propria and a predominantly polymorphonuclear infiltrate.

❑ **103** Is postulated to be due to a local butyrate deficiency.

❑ **104** Is typically associated with flask-shaped ulcers.

❑ **105** Is associated with characteristic yellow/grey plaques on sigmoidoscopy.

Theme: Jaundice

A Prehepatic jaundice
B Hepatic jaundice
C Posthepatic jaundice

Select the most likely type of jaundice from the list above that would be indicated by the clinical findings or associated with the conditions listed below. Each option may be used once, more than once, or not at all.

❑ **106** Pruritus.

❑ **107** Intake of hepatotoxic drugs.

❑ **108** Incompatible blood transfusion.

❑ **109** Chlorpromazine-induced jaundice.

❑ **110** Chronic active hepatitis.

❑ **111** Halothane-induced jaundice.

❑ **112** Thalassaemia.

❑ **113** Sclerosing cholangitis.

❑ **114** Hepatic abscesses.

❑ **115** Rotor's syndrome.

Theme: Colorectal surgery

A Left hemicolectomy
B Transverse loop colostomy
C Anterior resection
D Panproctocolectomy
E Subtotal colectomy
F Abdominoperineal resection
G Ileocolonic bypass
H Hartmann's procedure
I Sigmoid colectomy and primary anastomosis

For each of the patients described below, select the most appropriate surgical option from the list above. Each option may be used once, more than once, or not at all.

❑ **116** A 55-year-old man reattends the surgical outpatient department with rectal bleeding. He has recently completed a course of chemoradiotherapy for a squamous anal carcinoma. He underwent an examination under anaesthesia (EUA) which revealed some residual tumour.

❑ **117** A 30-year-old woman with known ulcerative colitis is admitted as an emergency with abdominal distension, vomiting, rectal bleeding and dehydration. She undergoes a course of conservative medical management but does not respond to steroids and immunosuppressive therapy. Her albumin level is 20 g/l, WBC 25×10^9/l and her colonic diameter on AXR is 9 cm.

❑ **118** A 45-year-old man is admitted as an emergency to the A&E department with generalised peritonitis. Following aggressive resuscitation he is taken to the operating theatre where a hard 4-cm mass in the sigmoid colon is found. There is gross faecal contamination of the peritoneal cavity. His liver has one umbilicated nodule in the left lobe. The rest of the laparotomy is normal.

Theme: Anatomy of the urogenital system

A Uterus
B Round ligament of the ovary
C Urethra
D Bladder
E Vas deferens
F Suspensory ligament of the ovary
G Testis
H Perineal membrane

For each of the statements below, select the most likely option from the list above. Each option may be used once, more than once, or not at all.

❑ **119** Lies superior to the ureter.

❑ **120** Transmits the ovarian vessels.

❑ **121** Has an internal sphincter that contracts during ejaculation.

❑ **122** Transmits the dorsal vein of the penis.

❑ **123** Is separated from the rectum by peritoneum.

❑ **124** Attaches the ovary to the uterus.

❑ **125** Intervenes between the uterus and pubic symphysis.

PRACTICE PAPER 2 – MULTIPLE CHOICE QUESTIONS

Time allowed: 2½ hrs

1 Associated features of rheumatoid arthritis include

- ❑ A Heberden's nodes
- ❑ B synovitis
- ❑ C normal ESR
- ❑ D early joint destruction
- ❑ E periarticular erosions

2 Bladder calculi

- ❑ A are usually secondary to bladder outlet obstruction
- ❑ B are associated with upper urinary tract calculi in 15–20% of cases
- ❑ C are most commonly composed of calcium oxalate
- ❑ D usually present with obstructive rather than irritative symptoms
- ❑ E can be diagnosed by a simple urine test

3 The middle ear

- ❑ A has the facial nerve running through its roof
- ❑ B is lined with a mucous membrane
- ❑ C contains all the auditory ossicles
- ❑ D has the internal carotid artery running anterior
- ❑ E has a promontory in the projection of the lateral semicircular canal
- ❑ F has the internal jugular vein running medial

4 Traumatic rupture of the oesophagus

- ❑ A may produce mediastinal emphysema
- ❑ B may result in mediastinitis if left untreated
- ❑ C is most easily diagnosed by oesophagoscopy
- ❑ D when associated with blunt trauma is known as Boerhaave's syndrome
- ❑ E when due to upper GI endoscopy usually occurs at the gastro-oesophageal junction

5 The palatine tonsillar bed

- ❑ A lies in the oral cavity
- ❑ B is floored by the middle constrictor muscle
- ❑ C contains the superior pharyngeal nerve
- ❑ D is pierced by branches of the facial artery
- ❑ E is drained by the external palatine vein

6 Causes of massive splenomegaly include

- ❑ A Chagas' disease
- ❑ B malaria
- ❑ C chronic hepatitis C
- ❑ D chronic myeloid leukaemia
- ❑ E myelofibrosis

7 Keloid scars

- ❑ A are treated by triamcinolone injections
- ❑ B may occur on mucosal surfaces
- ❑ C should be treated by surgery
- ❑ D rarely occurs in the mid-sternal region
- ❑ E should be treated by radiotherapy
- ❑ F are reduced along Langer's lines
- ❑ G may give rise to contractures across joint lines

8 The following are recognised surgical treatments for lymphoedema:

- ❑ A Homan's operation
- ❑ B lymphovenous microanastomosis
- ❑ C long saphenous vein transplantation
- ❑ D Trendelenburg's operation
- ❑ E mesenteric bridge operation

9 A term infant weighing 3.1 kg

- ❑ A requires about 450 ml of formula milk daily for adequate fluid and calories
- ❑ B should be maintained on 700 ml of normal saline per day intravenously
- ❑ C is at high risk of necrotising enterocolitis
- ❑ D is at risk of developing hypoglycaemia postoperatively
- ❑ E should pass meconium in the first 24 hours after birth

10 The ischiorectal fossae

- ❑ A communicate across the midline
- ❑ B contain the inferior rectal branches of the pudendal nerve
- ❑ C have a base formed by skin
- ❑ D have anterior recesses above the perineal membrane
- ❑ E contain the internal pudendal vessels

11 Acute septic arthritis of the knee

- ❑ A is most commonly caused by *Streptococcus* spp.
- ❑ B is initially managed by aspiration and culture of the fluid from the knee
- ❑ C should be managed with non-weight-bearing for 4–6 weeks
- ❑ D may cause locking
- ❑ E may lead to secondary osteoarthritis

12 Associated features of familial adenomatous polyposis (FAP) include

- ❑ A atrophic gastritis
- ❑ B gastric adenomas
- ❑ C duodenal adenomas
- ❑ D uveitis
- ❑ E medullary thyroid cancer

13 In the gluteal region, the sciatic nerve lies

- ❑ A on the piriformis muscle
- ❑ B deep in the upper outer quadrant
- ❑ C on the capsule of the hip joint
- ❑ D medial to the inferior gluteal vessels
- ❑ E anterior to the obturator internus muscle

14 Intimate relations of the left recurrent laryngeal nerve include the

- ❑ A oesophagus
- ❑ B trachea
- ❑ C left subclavian artery
- ❑ D ligamentum arteriosum
- ❑ E inferior thyroid artery

15 Sigmoid volvulus

- ❑ A is seen most frequently in the sixth and seventh decades of life
- ❑ B is a rare cause of colonic obstruction in Africans
- ❑ C is associated with a long, narrow, sigmoid mesenteric attachment
- ❑ D usually twists in a clockwise direction
- ❑ E is more common than caecal volvulus

16 The right renal artery

- ❑ A branches several times before entering the kidney
- ❑ B gives a branch to the ureter
- ❑ C lies anterior to the renal vein
- ❑ D lies anterior to the IVC

17 Acute appendicitis

- ❑ A has a peak incidence in the fourth decade
- ❑ B may cause microscopic haematuria
- ❑ C usually presents with vomiting followed by abdominal pain
- ❑ D may cause diarrhoea
- ❑ E complicated by an appendix mass, should initially be treated conservatively

18 In Hirschsprung's disease

- ❑ A there is absent sympathetic nerve supply to the bowel
- ❑ B there is frequent distal rectal sparing
- ❑ C there is a male predominance
- ❑ D the lumen of the aganglionic segment is grossly dilated
- ❑ E enterocolitis may be a complication

19 Perforated duodenal ulcer

- ❑ A is normally situated posteriorly
- ❑ B can be treated conservatively with antibiotics
- ❑ C is usually found in the second part of the duodenum
- ❑ D may be repaired by an omental patch
- ❑ E may be treated by a partial gastrectomy

20 Inflammatory bowel disease (IBD)

- ❑ A Crohn's disease has a much higher prevalence than ulcerative colitis in Western populations
- ❑ B the number of cases has risen over the past four decades
- ❑ C is most common in early adult life
- ❑ D has a higher prevalence in the lower social classes
- ❑ E has a higher incidence in Jews living outside Israel

21 The ureter

- ❑ A is supplied by lumbar arteries
- ❑ B lies anterior to the gonadal vessels
- ❑ C is crossed anteriorly by the vas deferens
- ❑ D lies over the external iliac artery in its distal third
- ❑ E has a nerve supply to its upper third from the T10 segment of the spinal cord

22 At the knee joint

- ❑ A the popliteus tendon is intracapsular
- ❑ B the suprapatellar bursa communicates with the joint
- ❑ C the iliotibial tract inserts into the fibula
- ❑ D the anterior cruciate ligament is supplied by the middle geniculate artery
- ❑ E rotation occurs below the menisci

23 Colorectal carcinoma is

- ❑ A the second commonest cause of cancer death in the UK
- ❑ B the second commonest cancer in the UK
- ❑ C usually inherited
- ❑ D three times commoner in first-degree relatives than the normal population
- ❑ E commoner in Africa

24 Thyrotoxicosis

❑ A is often caused by 'hot' nodules
❑ B is usually caused by elevated immunoglobulins
❑ C is associated with increased appetite and weight
❑ D may present with pretibial myxoedema
❑ E has an equal sex distribution

25 Congenital dislocation of the hip

❑ A is more common in boys
❑ B is most commonly bilateral
❑ C is associated with acetabular dysplasia
❑ D should initially be investigated by ultrasound
❑ E may present in adulthood

26 Aortic dissection

❑ A can present as a stroke
❑ B may result in paraplegia
❑ C requires immediate restoration of circulating blood volume
❑ D can be diagnosed correctly in 85% of cases by CT scan
❑ E typically presents with profound hypotension

27 The trigeminal nerve

❑ A supplies the buccinator muscle
❑ B supplies the muscles of mastication
❑ C the ophthalmic and maxillary divisions of which are only sensory
❑ D is sensory to the temporomandibular joint
❑ E supplies sensation to the angle of the mandible

28 Anal fissures

❑ A when chronic may be healed by glyceryl trinitrate (GTN) in 90% of cases
❑ B may be treated by a partial surgical division of the external sphincter
❑ C are associated with constipated stool
❑ D are most common in the third and fourth decades of life
❑ E often cause bleeding

29 The following tumours are associated with the given risk factors:

- ❑ A scrotal carcinoma and chimney sweeps
- ❑ B bladder cancer and dye workers
- ❑ C renal transitional-cell carcinoma and phenacetin abuse
- ❑ D penile cancer and circumcision
- ❑ E prostate cancer and vasectomy

30 Cervical rib

- ❑ A most commonly produces arterial symptoms
- ❑ B may produce a bruit in the supraclavicular fossa
- ❑ C causes paraesthesia most commonly in the C6 nerve root distribution
- ❑ D is bilateral in 50% of cases
- ❑ E is not associated with arm swelling

31 Secondary haemorrhage

- ❑ A occurs within 24 hours
- ❑ B may be massive
- ❑ C usually requires a blood transfusion
- ❑ D is associated with a deep infection
- ❑ E is the result of anticoagulation

32 Recognised causes of Raynaud's syndrome include

- ❑ A phenoxybenzamine
- ❑ B cryoglobinaemia
- ❑ C rheumatoid arthritis
- ❑ D Horner's syndrome
- ❑ E cervical rib

33 Anorectal lesions associated with HIV-infected patients include

- ❑ A Kaposi's sarcoma
- ❑ B apocrine hydrocystoma
- ❑ C rectal ulceration
- ❑ D lymphoma
- ❑ E neurofibromas

34 The base of the bladder lies on the

- ❑ A seminal vesicles
- ❑ B ureters
- ❑ C ductus (vas) deferens
- ❑ D anterior vaginal wall
- ❑ E cervix

35 A fall in serum calcium levels causes

- ❑ A reduced osteoclastic activity
- ❑ B increased vitamin D production
- ❑ C increased bone resorption
- ❑ D reduced parathyroid hormone (PTH) secretion
- ❑ E renal tubule impermeability to calcium

36 Posterior relations of the right kidney include the

- ❑ A psoas muscle
- ❑ B subcostal nerve
- ❑ C peritoneum
- ❑ D diaphragm
- ❑ E right suprarenal gland

37 Faecal occult blood tests (guaiac-based)

- ❑ A can detect blood loss of less than 0.5 ml/day
- ❑ B rarely give rise to false-positive results
- ❑ C are unaffected by the anatomical level of bleeding
- ❑ D may be positive whilst taking oral iron
- ❑ E are unaffected by faecal rehydration

38 Surgical anatomy of the thyroid gland

- ❑ A the thyroid gland has a definite fine capsule
- ❑ B Berry's ligament connects the thyroid to the cricoid cartilage and upper trachea
- ❑ C the inferior parathyroid glands are more constant in position than the superior parathyroid glands
- ❑ D the middle thyroid veins are more constant in position than the superior and inferior thyroid veins
- ❑ E unilateral recurrent laryngeal nerve division results in the contralateral vocal cord lying in the mid or cadaveric position

39 Infantile hypertrophic pyloric stenosis

- ❑ A has an approximate incidence of 3:1000 live births
- ❑ B is associated with bile-stained vomiting
- ❑ C has no known familial association
- ❑ D does not occur in premature babies
- ❑ E requires a test feed to palpate the classical 'olive'

40 The following drugs may be used in the treatment of benign prostatic hypertrophy:

- ❑ A tamsulosin
- ❑ B alfuzosin
- ❑ C tolterodine
- ❑ D finasteride
- ❑ E goserelin

41 Transection of the cervical part of the sympathetic chain at the root of the neck results in

- ❑ A vasomotor changes in the arm
- ❑ B ptosis
- ❑ C pupillary dilatation
- ❑ D ablation of sympathetic supply to the pulmonary plexus
- ❑ E loss of sweating over the C4 dermatome

42 Congenital diaphragmatic hernia

- ❑ A defect is most commonly anteromedial
- ❑ B mostly occurs on the left
- ❑ C commonly presents with neonatal respiratory distress
- ❑ D can be diagnosed on plain chest X-ray
- ❑ E is associated with other anomalies in about 10% of cases
- ❑ F if uncorrected can lead to persistent fetal circulation

43 Slipped femoral epiphysis

- ❑ A may be complicated by avascular necrosis of the femoral head
- ❑ B may lead to coxa valga
- ❑ C is more common in boys
- ❑ D commonly occurs at the age of 5 years
- ❑ E is usually caused by a single traumatic event

44 Abdominal aortic aneurysms

- ❑ A are associated with visible calcification on plain abdominal X-rays in 60% of cases
- ❑ B may be caused by *Salmonella* spp.
- ❑ C are frequently caused by fungi
- ❑ D expand at a rate of 4 mm per year
- ❑ E measuring 7.5 cm in diameter have a 5-year rupture rate of 45%

45 The trachea

- ❑ A begins at the level of the thyroid cartilage
- ❑ B is in contact with the right pleura
- ❑ C has fibroelastic cartilage in its wall
- ❑ D is innervated by the recurrent laryngeal nerve
- ❑ E is in contact with the left common carotid

46 Primary peritonitis

- ❑ A is usually caused by haematogenous spread of a single type of bacterium
- ❑ B has a strong association with cirrhosis of the liver
- ❑ C is associated with an ascitic eosinophilia
- ❑ D has a strong association with nephrosis
- ❑ E is most commonly caused by a Gram-positive coccus

47 Carcinoid tumours

- ❑ A are most commonly found in the large bowel
- ❑ B of the small bowel are most frequently found in the ileum
- ❑ C of the large bowel are most frequently found in the caecum
- ❑ D in the small bowel are often multiple
- ❑ E of the appendix are usually benign

48 Testicular seminoma is

- ❑ A a recognised cause of gynaecomastia
- ❑ B usually diagnosed by needle biopsy
- ❑ C radio-resistant
- ❑ D resistant to chemotherapy
- ❑ E associated with a disease-free survival rate of 99% for stage 1 disease

49 Hydatid disease of the liver

- ❑ A is caused by *Echinococcus granulosus*
- ❑ B may cause peritonitis
- ❑ C is successfully treated with metronidazole
- ❑ D is known to fistulate into the lung
- ❑ E is associated with pancytopenia

50 The prostate gland

- ❑ A is pierced by the ducts of the seminal vesicles
- ❑ B has a venous plexus contained within its capsule
- ❑ C lies below the urogenital diaphragm
- ❑ D contains the membranous urethra
- ❑ E is separated from the rectum by peritoneum

51 Relations of the pituitary include the

- ❑ A diaphragma sellae
- ❑ B optic chiasma
- ❑ C sphenoid sinus
- ❑ D temporal lobe
- ❑ E cavernous sinus

52 At the ankle joint the

- ❑ A peroneus tertius tendon grooves the lateral malleolus
- ❑ B flexor digitorum longus tendon grooves the medial malleolus
- ❑ C deltoid ligament is attached to the calcaneus
- ❑ D posterior tibial artery lies between the tibialis posterior and flexor digitorum longus tendons
- ❑ E tibial nerve lies anterior to the posterior tibial artery

53 A below-knee amputation

- ❑ A should have no prosthesis fitted for at least 6 weeks
- ❑ B should be placed in plaster of Paris postoperatively
- ❑ C is an 'end-stump'
- ❑ D stump continues to shrink for 6 months postoperatively

54 The following structures are normally encountered during dissection for a right hemicolectomy:

❑ A caudate lobe
❑ B inferior vena cava
❑ C third part of the duodenum
❑ D right ureter
❑ E gonadal vessels

55 Exomphalos

❑ A has an incidence of 1 in 5000
❑ B is associated with major abnormalities in 10% of cases
❑ C is associated with the Beckwith–Wiedemann syndrome
❑ D can lead to respiratory distress when primary reduction and closure is carried out
❑ E is a sac made of the amniotic membrane and peritoneum

56 Pancreatic carcinoma

❑ A 40% of cases arise in the neck of the pancreas
❑ B is better visualised with CT than by transabdominal ultrasound
❑ C has typical radiological features on ERCP
❑ D invading the portal vein precludes resection

57 The Eustachian tube

❑ A drains the inner ear
❑ B pierces the pharyngobasilar fascia
❑ C gives attachment to the tensor veli palatini muscle
❑ D can be obstructed by an enlarging palatine tonsil
❑ E closes during swallowing

58 In the female reproductive tract

❑ A the ovarian artery supplies the fallopian tube
❑ B most of the anterior surface of the uterus is covered by peritoneum
❑ C ureteric calculi are palpable per vaginum
❑ D the ovary lies posterior to the broad ligament
❑ E lymph drains from the uterine tubes to the superficial inguinal lymph nodes
❑ F the major arterial supply of the uterus originates from the internal iliac artery
❑ G the suspensory ligament of the ovary is a remnant of the gubernaculum

59 Scaphoid fractures

❑ A are prone to causing avascular necrosis in the distal fragment
❑ B their treatment involves an immobilising cast that includes the forearm, wrist and whole thumb
❑ C may require operative reduction when the fracture is displaced
❑ D often produces tenderness in the anatomical snuffbox
❑ E are most common in elderly women

60 Intussusception

❑ A is more common in males
❑ B is more common in the winter months
❑ C a Meckel's diverticulum is the most common pathological lead-point
❑ D the advancing telescoping inner segment is defined as the intussuscipiens
❑ E 'redcurrant jelly' stools are seen in 80% of cases

61 Obstructive jaundice is associated with

❑ A delayed wound healing
❑ B increased sepsis
❑ C increased incidence of DVT
❑ D renal failure
❑ E increased bleeding due to a raised prothrombin time

62 The facial nerve supplies the

❑ A stapedius
❑ B buccinator
❑ C medial pterygoid
❑ D parasympathetics to the lacrimal gland
❑ E parasympathetics to the parotid gland

63 Paget's disease of bone

❑ A is associated with sarcomatous change in 5% of cases
❑ B can be associated with cardiac complications
❑ C shows a decreased alkaline phosphatase level
❑ D affects men more commonly than women
❑ E usually affects the upper limb girdle

64 Indications for carotid endarterectomy include

❑ A symptomatic, severe (>70%), carotid artery stenosis
❑ B symptomatic, moderate (30–69%), carotid artery stenosis
❑ C symptomatic, mild (<30%), carotid artery stenosis
❑ D large, completed ischaemic stroke within the preceding year
❑ E TIA sustained 2 years ago attributed to carotid artery stenosis

65 Hernias of the groin

❑ A indirect inguinal hernias enter through the internal inguinal ring medial to the inferior epigastric vessels
❑ B direct inguinal hernias usually emerge through the lateral aspect of the posterior wall of the inguinal canal
❑ C sliding hernias have small bowel forming part of the wall of the sac
❑ D femoral hernias are more common than inguinal hernias in women
❑ E enlarging femoral hernias pass through the saphenous opening of the fascia lata, over the inguinal ligament, and into the subcutaneous tissues superficial to Scarpa's fascia

PRACTICE PAPER 2 – EXTENDED MATCHING QUESTIONS

Theme: Spinal pathology

A Acute disc prolapse
B Scheuermann's disease
C TB of the spine
D Spondylolisthesis

For each of the patients listed below, select the diagnosis that best explains the clinical situation from the list above. Each option may be used once, more than once, or not at all.

❑ **66** An 18-year-old fast bowler and keen athlete, presents with pain when extending his hip, he walks with scoliosis – acute onset.

❑ **67** A young immigrant from Bangladesh presents with lower back pain and fever.

Theme: Nerve damage

A Horner's syndrome
B Posterior interosseus nerve lesion
C Neurapraxia of the median nerve
D Neurapraxia of the common peroneal nerve
E Neurotmesis of the common peroneal nerve
F Sciatic nerve injury
G Neurapraxia of the radial nerve
H Neurotmesis of the medial nerve

For each of the patients listed below, select the site and type of nerve damage that best explains the clinical situation from the list above. Each option may be used once, more than once, or not at all.

❑ **68** A 21-year-old man sustained a comminuted fracture of the right femur and a fracture of the ipsilateral tibia and fibula. He was treated with skeletal traction and a below-knee plaster overnight. On review it was noticed that he could not dorsiflex his right toes.

❑ **69** A child falls on an outstretched hand and sustains a severely displaced supracondylar fracture of the humerus.

❑ **70** Following a difficult elective plating of a non-union fracture of the humeral shaft, the patient was unable to extend his fingers and wrist. No nerves were visualised during the procedure.

❑ **71** A motorcyclist came off his bike at considerable speed. Both he and his bike were then dragged down the road by a car. On examination he had a flail left upper limb.

❑ **72** Following a total hip replacement performed via a posterior approach, the patient was noted to have a foot drop.

Theme: Knee injuries

A Injury to the medial meniscus
B Anterior cruciate rupture
C Patellar fracture
D Haemarthrosis
E Medial ligament rupture
F Tibial plateau fracture

For each of the clinical situations described below, select the most likely diagnosis from the list above. Each option may be used once, more than once, or not at all.

❑ **73** A 29-year-old man was hit by a car as he ran across the road. He was subsequently unable to weight-bear. His knee was bruised, swollen and tender.

❑ **74** A 45-year-old woman stumbled over an uneven paving stone and landed heavily on her knee. She walked aided into A&E with a swollen painful knee and was unable to straight-leg raise.

❑ **75** A footballer sustained a twisting injury to his flexed knee whilst playing a game yesterday. He was unable to complete the game and by this morning his knee was very swollen. He was unable to fully flex or extend his knee.

❑ **76** A 25-year-old man landed awkwardly having jumped for a ball in the line-out during a rugby match. He heard a pop, and was unable to complete the game. He noticed his knee swell immediately.

❑ **77** A 25-year-old man was involved in a tackle during a football game today. A valgus force was applied to the knee – he fell to the ground and noted that his knee was at a 'funny angle'. He has been unable to weight-bear and says that his knee feels 'unsafe'. On examination, his knee is generally tender, there is significant laxity on valgus stress but no definite effusion.

Theme: Paediatric newborn gastrointestinal disorders

A Hirschsprung's disease
B Intussusception
C Meconium ileus
D Duodenal atresia
E Necrotising enterocolitis
F Pyloric stenosis
G Biliary atresia

For each of the patients described below, select the most likely diagnosis from the list of options above. Each option may be used once, more than once, or not at all.

❑ **78** A 3-day-old child presents with a scaphoid abdomen, and is unable to feed with bilious vomiting.

❑ **79** A 10-day-old child presents with a right abdominal mass and distension, with a history of passing meconium for only 3 days with the help of suppositories. He is now passing blood per rectum.

❑ **80** A baby presents needing enemas to open its bowels owing to a 24-hour delay in passing meconium.

Theme: Thyroid disease

A Subtotal thyroidectomy
B Hemithyroidectomy
C Total thyroidectomy
D Radio-iodine treatment
E Enucleation

From the options above, select the most appropriate treatment for the patients below. Each option may be used once, more than once, or not at all.

❑ **81** A 25-year-old woman with Grave's disease is thyrotoxic. Medical treatment has failed to control her symptoms and she is hoping to start a family in the next few years.

❑ **82** A 55-year-old woman presents with a swelling in her thyroid. Investigations has revealed it to be a lymphoma.

❑ **83** A 45-year-old man presented with a lump in the right lobe of his thyroid. Fine-needle aspiration revealed it to be follicular in nature.

Theme: Parathyroid glands

A Inferior parathyroid glands
B Superior parathyroid glands

For each of the statements below, select the correct anatomical structure from the list above. Each option may be used once, more than once, or not at all.

❑ **84** Mostly lie adjacent to the cricothyroid notch close to the recurrent laryngeal nerve.

❑ **85** When ectopic, usually lie in the posterior mediastinum.

❑ **86** Are derived from the third branchial pouch.

❑ **87** May lie anywhere from the mandible to the anterior mediastinum.

❑ **88** Are derived from the fourth branchial pouch.

❑ **89** 20% lie on or within the suprasternal portion of the thymus.

Theme: Lymphatic drainage

A Internal iliac lymph nodes
B Para-aortic lymph nodes
C Deep inguinal lymph nodes
D Superficial inguinal lymph nodes
E Superior mesenteric lymph nodes

For each of the anatomical areas below, select the most likely group of lymph nodes these areas would first drain from the list above. Each option may be used once only, more than once, or not at all.

❑ **90** Testes
❑ **91** Scrotum
❑ **92** Vulva
❑ **93** Base of cervix
❑ **94** Distal rectum
❑ **95** Big toe

Theme: Surface/radiological anatomy of the anterior abdominal wall

A Transpyloric plane
B L4 vertebral body
C L5 vertebral body
D Mid-inguinal point
E Above and medial to the pubic tubercle
F Sacroiliac joint
G Below and lateral to the pubic tubercle
H Midpoint of inguinal ligament
I Umbilicus
J 12th rib
K 10th rib
L Transtubercular plane

For each of the statements below, select the most likely option from the list above. Each option may be used once, more than once, or not at all.

❑ **96** External ring of the femoral canal.

❑ **97** Termination of the spinal cord in adults.

❑ **98** Spleen.

Theme: Hernias

A Epigastric hernia
B Spigelian hernia
C Obturator hernia
D Lumbar hernia
E Gluteal hernia
F Sciatic hernia
G Perineal hernia
H Diaphragmatic hernia

For each site of herniation below, select the most likely hernial type from the list above. Each answer may be used once, more than once, or not at all.

❑ **99** Linea alba

❑ **100** Obturator canal

❑ **101** Lesser sciatic notch

Theme: Surgical investigations

A Gastrografin enema
B Abdominal CT scan
C small bowel follow-through
D ERCP
E Abdominal ultrasound
F Barium enema (double-contrast)
G Colonoscopy

For each of the following scenarios, select the most appropriate investigation from the list above. Each option may be used once, more than once, or not at all.

❑ **102** Hepatic hydatid cyst.

❑ **103** Uncomplicated diverticular disease of the colon.

❑ **104** Sclerosing cholangitis.

❑ **105** Choledocholithiasis.

Theme: Abdominal pain investigations (diagnostic)

A FBC
B Serum amylase
C Erect chest X-ray
D Supine abdominal X-ray
E Angiography (mesenteric)
F CT
G Barium enema
H Barium meal and follow-through
I Abdominal ultrasound

For each of the patients described below, select the most likely investigation from the list of options above. Each option may be used once, more than once, or not at all.

❑ **106** A 75-year-old female orthopaedic patient on steroids for COPD and diclofenac for pain presents with acute, sudden-onset epigastric pain.

❑ **107** A 70-year-old psychiatric patient presents with periumbilical discomfort, gross abdominal distension and absolute constipation but no vomiting.

❑ **108** A 34-year-old woman with severe asthma was started on steroids. She later presents with acute-onset epigastric pain and vomiting. On examination she has decreased bowel sounds, guarding and rigidity.

Theme: Anatomy of the posterior abdominal wall

A Kidney
B Psoas major muscle
C Lumbar plexus
D Ureter
E Sympathetic trunk
F Ilioinguinal nerve
G Bare area of the liver
H Superior rectal artery

For each of the statements below, select the most likely option from the list above. Each option may be used once, more than once, or not at all.

❑ **109** Lies medial to the left ureter.

❑ **110** Is embedded in the psoas major muscle.

❑ **111** Lies anterior to the subcostal vessels.

❑ **112** Contacts the right suprarenal gland.

Theme: Renal physiology

A Distal convoluted tubule
B Proximal convoluted tubule
C Descending limb of loop of Henle
D Ascending limb of loop of Henle
E Collecting ducts

For each of the statements below, select the most likely option from the list above. Each option may be used once, more than once, or not at all.

❑ **113** Site of facultative potassium control.

❑ **114** Main site of glucose reabsorption.

❑ **115** Main site of sodium reabsorption.

❑ **116** Generation of hyperosmolality of renal medullary interstitium.

Theme: Anatomy of the pelvic vasculature

A Superior gluteal artery
B Superior vesical artery
C Gonadal veins
D Superior rectal vein
E Inferior vesical artery
F Lateral sacral veins
G Internal iliac artery
H Uterine artery

For each of the statements below, select the most likely option from the list above. Each option may be used once, more than once, or not at all.

❑ **117** Accompanies the ureter.

❑ **118** Drains the middle third of the ureters.

❑ **119** Is a branch of the posterior division of the internal iliac artery.

❑ **120** Runs in the transverse cervical ligament (cardinal).

Theme: 5-year graft patency rates

A Reversed vein femoropopliteal graft
B Femoropopliteal PTFE graft patency (below knee)
C Aortobifemoral graft
D Axillofemoral graft
E Femoral–femoral crossover graft

For each of the percentages below, select the most likely single graft from the options listed above. Each option may be used once, more than once, or not at all.

❑ **121** 70%

❑ **122** 80%

❑ **123** 60%

❑ **124** 35%

❑ **125** 90%

ANSWERS – CHAPTER 1: LOCOMOTOR

1.1 Peripheral nerve anatomy

1. E Common peroneal
2. C Obturator
3. J S1 nerve root
4. G Sciatic

The most common lower limb neural injury is to the common peroneal nerve, either by direct trauma or by pressure from a plaster cast at the neck of the fibula. Common presentations include 'foot drop' (paralysis of the extensor muscles supplied by the deep peroneal branch) and inversion of the foot (less obvious because there is paralysis of the peroneus longus and brevis muscles – superficial peroneal nerve and the tibialis anterior muscles are also paralysed – deep peroneal nerve). Thus, only the inverting action of the tibialis posterior is present.

Anaesthesia over the lower lateral calf and dorsum of the foot is also seen (superficial peroneal nerve). Note that branches of the lateral cutaneous nerve of the calf arise from the common peroneal nerve above the lesion in the popliteal fossa and, thus, sensation over the upper lateral skin of the calf is preserved.

Pelvic pathology may present with referred pain over the cutaneous distribution of the obturator nerve, because the lateral pelvic peritoneum is supplied by this nerve as it passes retroperitoneally through the pelvis. An ovarian tumour growing out from the posterior surface of the broad ligament into the rectouterine pouch might irritate the peritoneum of the lateral pelvic wall.

L5/S1 disc prolapse would damage the S1 spinal nerve. The L5 spinal nerve escapes injury because it exits the spinal canal above the prolapse in the L5 intervertebral canal. The sciatic nerve may be injured in 20% of fracture dislocations of the hip, since it passes over the posterior aspect of the joint capsule. As a result, all flexors and extensors below the knee are paralysed and all skin is anaesthetic except for those areas innervated by the saphenous (medial calf and medial foot) and posterior cutaneous nerve of the thigh (upper posterior aspect of the calf). Paralysis of the hamstring muscles would also occur.

1.2 ABDE

The femoral (Scarpa's) triangle is a fascial space in the upper medial thigh. Its sides are formed superiorly by the inguinal ligament, medially by the adductor longus and laterally by the sartorius. The floor is formed by the iliopsoas, pectineus and adductor longus. The triangle contains the femoral vessels and nerve. Within the femoral triangle, the femoral artery divides into its deep and superficial branches; and the femoral vein receives deep femoral and saphenous tributaries.

1.3 ACE

The greater sciatic notch is converted into the greater sciatic foramen by the sacrospinous ligament, and transmits many structures between the gluteal and pelvic regions. This includes: superior and inferior gluteal vessels and nerves; sciatic nerve; posterior cutaneous nerve of the thigh; the nerve to obturator internus and quadratus femoris; the pudendal nerve; and the internal pudendal vessels. The lesser sciatic foramen is the space between the sacrospinous and sacrotuberous ligaments. It contains: the pudendal nerve; nerve and tendon to obturator internus; and the internal pudendal vessels.

The pudendal nerve and the internal pudendal vessels exit the pelvis via the greater sciatic foramen and enter the perineum through the lesser sciatic foramen. Similarly, the nerve to the obturator internus leaves the pelvis via the greater sciatic foramen and soon re-enters the pelvis through the lesser sciatic foramen.

1.4 Calcium homeostasis

1. D Hypocalciuric hypercalcaemia

2. B Secondary hyperparathyroidism

3. A Primary hyperparathyroidism

Parathyroid (PTH) hormone acts on bones producing osteoclastic resorption so elevating the plasma calcium. PTH also acts on the kidney by increasing calcium reabsorption, decreasing phosphate reabsorption and causing elevation of 25-hydroxycholecalciferol. Despite this, hypercalciuria usually results from elevated levels of PTH. The normal urinary calcium is 2.5–7.5 mmol/day.

Familial hypocalciuric hypercalcaemia (FHH) is a rare condition (often appears in exams). In FHH, a high plasma calcium is sensed by the parathyroid glands as normal. The patient therefore has hypercalcaemia with normal PTH levels. They require no treatment.

1.5 ACD

The femoral sheath is a downward continuation of the abdominal fascia about 2.5 cm below the inguinal ligament. It is believed to allow for femoral vessel movement in the inguinal region during movement of the hip. The mnemonic 'NAVEL' describes some of the key structures in this region (from lateral to medial): femoral **n**erve, **a**rtery, **v**ein, **e**mpty space, **l**ymphatics (i.e. Cloquet's). Apart from the femoral nerve that lies most lateral, all the other structures in the mnemonic are encased in the femoral sheath. The mentioned empty space and lymphatic compartments form the 'femoral canal' where femoral hernias may occur. Therefore, the femoral canal is in the most medial portion of the femoral sheath. The femoral ring is the abdominal opening into the femoral canal. At 2–3 cm below the inguinal ligament, the femoral sheath fuses with the adventitia of the femoral vessels. The pubic branch of the inferior epigastric artery replaces the obturator artery in about 30% of cases, and may be at risk in a femoral hernia repair.

1.6 BD

The Trendelenburg test is used to assess stability of the hip. A positive Trendelenburg test is seen with any painful disorder of the hip. It is also present with a dislocated or subluxed hip and in other conditions where the proximal femoral anatomy is abnormal (short femoral neck with high-riding trochanter). Weak abductor muscles will also lead to a positive test. The abductors of the hip include piriformis, gluteus medius and minimis. Pectineus adducts the hip. The other adductors of the hip are gracilis, adductor longus, brevis and magnus.

1.7 Shoulder pain

1. B Supraspinatus rupture
2. A Supraspinatus tendonitis
3. E Acromioclavicular joint dislocation
4. D Biceps rupture
5. F Posterior dislocation of the shoulder (and G frozen shoulder)

A complete tear of the supraspinatus tendon may occur after a long period of chronic tendinitis. Active abduction is impossible and any attempt produces a characteristic shrug; however, passive abduction is full and once the arm has been raised to beyond 90°, the patient maintains arm elevation using the deltoid muscle. This is known as the 'abduction paradox'.

Supraspinatus tendinitis usually occurs in a patient <40 years of age. The typical history is development of shoulder pain after vigorous/ strenuous exercise. On active abduction, scapulohumeral movement is disturbed and pain is aggravated as the arm traverses an arc between 60 and 120°. An acute calcific tendonitis may develop in response to 'overuse' and may present with excruciating pain. Such acute symptoms arising from a joint should also raise the possibility of a septic arthritis.

A direct blow to the shoulder may fracture the clavicle or cause disruption of the acromioclavicular joint. A palpable step can usually be felt, but this may be difficult as a result of swelling.

In the older patient, an acute tendon rupture can occur relatively easily and may affect tendons such as the biceps, quadriceps, Achilles or supraspinatus.

Epileptic fits can lead to posterior dislocation of the shoulder, which if missed results in a stiff and painful shoulder with the arm 'fixed' in internal rotation. Progressive pain and stiffness of the shoulder may also indicate a frozen shoulder.

1.8 Anatomy of the joints in the upper limb

1. A Shoulder

2. G First carpometacarpal

3. C Superior radioulnar

4. H Acromioclavicular

The shoulder joint has the tendon of the long head of the biceps muscle (invested in synovial membrane) running over the head of the humerus to attach to the supraglenoid tubercle.

The first carpometacarpal joint is a saddle joint allowing flexion, abduction, adduction, extension, rotation and opposition.

The annular ligament holds the head of the radius against the radial notch of the ulna.

Movements at the acromioclavicular joint are the reciprocal of those at the sternoclavicular joint.

1.9 BDE

More than 90% of shoulder dislocations are anterior and the head is usually in the subcoracoid position. There is flattening of the contour of the shoulder and the arm is held in some abduction. Posterior shoulder dislocation is much less common but is usually seen following epileptic fits or electric shocks. Axillary nerve palsy may cause deltoid muscle atrophy and paraesthesia in the upper arm. Closed reduction is achieved by either the Hippocratic method or Kocher's manoeuvre.

1.10 DE

Compartment syndrome is caused by increased pressure within a closed myofascial compartment of a limb and may occur in the presence or absence of a fracture. The pressure increase is secondary to tissue oedema and/or haemorrhage. Unless the BP in the limb is low (due to haemorrhage or arterial obstruction) the pressure within the compartment rarely rises sufficiently to occlude the pulse distally. Thus loss of a peripheral pulse is a **very** late sign. The muscles in the involved compartment are ischaemic and this causes considerable pain on passive/active movement.

1.11 ABCD

Dupuytren's contracture is a thickening and fibrosis of the palmar fascia which may lead to a flexion contracture. This particularly affects the ring and little fingers of the hands with loss of function. In most cases the condition becomes bilateral. It may affect the foot and be associated with Peyronie's disease of the penis. Common conditions causing Dupuytren's contracture include cirrhosis, rheumatoid arthritis, familial cause, antiepileptic agents (phenytoin), trauma. An increase in oxygen free radicals in the fibrotic tissue has been noted. Treatment is by surgical excision of the involved fascia.

1.12 Bone pathology

1. E Avascular necrosis

2. D Bone cyst

Divers are at risk of caisson disease, which can produce avascular necrosis (AVN) of the humeral and femoral heads. However, the most common cause of AVN of the humeral head is steroid therapy.

The sclerotic edge at the fracture site indicates that the lesion is a bone cyst. Bone cysts tend to occur in the upper humerus, tibia and femur. Many disappear spontaneously, but they can be curetted and the cavity filled with bone chips.

1.13 AC

The blood supply of the femoral head is derived from three sources:

1. retinacular vessels running along the femoral neck under the joint capsule
2. via the nutrient artery into the medullary cavity
3. ligamentum teres (tiny proportion)

Displaced intracapsular fractures of the femoral neck are associated with damage to the two main supplies of blood to the femoral head. Thus, avascular necrosis is common and fracture union is unlikely. A hemiarthroplasty is the treatment of choice in the elderly patient. Cannulated screw fixation may be used in the young patient who has a relatively undisplaced femoral head and a recent onset of injury. Fracture of the upper femur is almost exclusively seen in elderly patients with bones weakened by osteoporosis. In impacted and minimally displaced fractures of the femoral neck, the fracture may be stable and it may be possible to weight-bear on the leg.

1.14 AB

The incidence of intracapsular fractures is increasing due to a rising elderly population. The mortality rate at 6 months can be as high as 40%. In displaced femoral neck fractures, the leg is shortened and externally rotated. The risk of avascular necrosis is related to the blood supply of the femoral head, being greater with intracapsular than extracapsular (intertrochanteric) fractures. Standard treatment is a hemiarthroplasty – the DHS is used for extracapsular fractures.

1.15 AE

Displaced intertrochanteric fractures cause shortening and external rotation of the leg. Adduction occurs due to the unopposed action of the adductors. Hemiarthroplasty is more frequently performed for intra-capsular fractures as the blood supply to the femoral head is more likely to be significantly compromised. In extracapsular fractures, the main blood supply is usually undisturbed and femoral head replacement is unnecessary. In such cases, DHS fixation is most frequently performed.

1.16 AE

Carpal tunnel syndrome is most frequently seen in women between 40 and 60 years of age. A multitude of conditions have been associated with carpal tunnel syndrome, including rheumatoid arthritis, myxoedema, nephrotic syndrome, acromegaly, multiple myeloma, amyloidosis, diabetes mellitus, alcoholism, haemophilia, pregnancy, gout and the menopause. Cervical spondylosis (degenerative change) may be associated with nerve root impingement, producing similar clinical features to carpal tunnel syndrome. Antiepileptic medication is associated with Dupuytren's contracture. Obesity is not by itself a risk factor. Wrist fractures associated with swelling and haematoma in the carpal tunnel cause acute compression of the median nerve – this is not usually seen with carpal bone injuries.

1.17 CD

Supracondylar fracture is one of the most common fractures in children and occurs much less frequently in the adult population. The cause is usually a fall on to the hand with the elbow flexed. The distal fragment may rarely be displaced anteriorly; the most common situation is for it to be displaced posteriorly. The elbow is swollen and the radial pulse may be absent if the brachial artery has been damaged by the fractured bone ends. Complications of this injury include: compartment syndrome; Volkmann's ischaemic contracture; neuropraxia to the median, ulnar and radial nerves; and malunion (cubitus varus). Wrist drop could be caused by damage to the radial but as muscular branches of the radial nerve leave the parent trunk proximally, the nerve to the wrist extensors will be well away from the main nerve trunk and well away from the site of injury in a supracondylar fracture.

1.18 Bone tumours

1. C Myeloma

2. A Osteosarcoma

3. D Osteochondroma

Myeloma is a malignant proliferation of plasma cells. One should suspect it in any patient with multiple lytic lesions and a high ESR. Renal failure is the usual cause of death.

Osteosarcoma occurs in 10–20-year-olds, but also has a second peak in the 7th decade, as it occurs in patients with Paget's disease. The overlying skin is often warm and shiny and radiographs may show periosteal elevation (Codman's angle) with sunray spicules. Osteosarcoma usually affects the distal femur, proximal tibia, proximal humerus and pelvis. Predisposing factors of osteosarcoma include radiotherapy, osteochondroma, fibrous dysplasia, osteopetrosis and bone infarct.

Ewing's sarcoma (children aged 5–15 years) is a tumour of vascular endothelium. It occurs in the diaphysis of long bones, and the periosteum has an onion-skin appearance due to lamellation. It may metastasise to other bones and the lungs.

1.19 BC

Flat feet are very common in children and individuals with ligamentous laxity. The condition has a familial tendency and is common to certain ethnic groups. Acquired flat foot may be due to dysfunction of the tibialis posterior tendon, secondary to trauma or inflammatory change. The vast majority of flat feet are pain-free and require no treatment. Orthotic supports are useful for the few feet that are painful. Painful flat feet may be treated by a triple fusion (subtalar, talonavicular and calcaneocuboid joints).

1.20 BD

Alcoholic polyneuropathy can occur in chronic alcoholics and is due to thiamine deficiency. Calf pain rather than foot pain is the common feature. Hallux rigidus is osteoarthritis of the first metatarsophalangeal joint and is commonly associated with significant pain and stiffness on exercise. An L2/L3 disc prolapse does not affect the foot but an L4/5 or L5/S1 lesion would. Rheumatoid arthritis by way of soft tissue or bony changes is a common cause of disabling pain. Dupuytren's contracture can affect the sole of the foot but the condition is not usually associated with pain.

1.21 ABE

Idiopathic (congenital) club feet are commoner in boys than girls and there is a familial tendency. Treatment begins at birth with stretching and strapping techniques. If surgical correction is required, this is usually done before the child starts to walk. Postural club foot is associated with oligohydramnios and usually resolves by the age of 3 months. Club feet may be associated with neuromuscular conditions such as spina bifida or syndromes such as arthrogryposis.

1.22 AD

The most likely diagnosis here would lie between an anterior cruciate ligament tear and a meniscal tear. The twisting nature of the injury is more suggestive of a meniscal injury. An anterior cruciate rupture frequently causes a 'popping' sound, producing a prominent haemarthrosis soon after the injury. Meniscal tears do not usually produce such a large effusion and the swelling comes on more slowly. Either a torn meniscus or ligament would cause soft tissue to impede movement of the knee joint, leading to a loss of full extension and/or full flexion. A locked knee is one that can flex but does not fully extend. This must be differentiated from a joint which has restricted movement due to pain.

A medial collateral ligament rupture is caused by a valgus force being applied to the knee. There may be considerable bleeding, but because of damage to the joint capsule itself there is rarely a localised effusion. Patella dislocation is usually associated with a sensation of the knee giving way and there is obvious deformity. Septic arthritis of the knee is associated with pain, swelling, tenderness and signs of inflammation. It may be precipitated by an episode of trauma, but this is more likely to be a minor injury rather than the one suggested by this scenario.

1.23 ACE

Tourniquets, even when used in an appropriate manner, will lead to vascular damage and thrombosis, soft tissue injury and nerve injury. It is important to record the time when the tourniquet is inflated. It should not remain constantly inflated for more than 2 hours. It is good practice to release the tourniquet before suturing the wound so as to identify the bleeding vessels and thus prevent postoperative haemorrhage. (An opposite point of view states that once the tourniquet is released the reactive hyperaemia in the limb leads to significant blood loss from a multitude of small vessels – this is mainly an orthopaedic point of view and it is good practice for surgical trainees to consider releasing the tourniquet before closure.) The tourniquet pressure should be just above arterial pressure otherwise bleeding would obscure the operating field.
A tourniquet must be used as part of the Biers' block technique or else toxic levels of local anaesthetic would reach into the general circulation.

1.24 BCDE

Steroids and diabetes mellitus increase the risk of wound infection and hence potential infection of joint replacement. The passage of a urinary catheter does cause a transient bacteraemia. If this is not covered with the appropriate antibiotic (such as gentamicin), deep-seated infection in the prosthesis may occur. Psoriasis leads to increased skin infections, and this itself is an independent risk factor.

1.25 BE

Young women with a valgus knee, ligamentous laxity and a deficient lateral femoral condyle are most at risk of having a dislocation of the patella. A weak vastus medialis is also a contributory factor.

1.26 ABE

Slipped upper femoral epiphysis is much more common in adolescent boys than girls and may present with knee pain rather than hip/groin pain. With a significant slip, the leg lies short and externally rotated. Severe acute (unstable) slips may lead to avascular necrosis of the femoral head. Treatment is by percutaneous pinning if the slip is moderate/minor – severe slips may require an osteotomy. The incidence of bilateral slips is difficult to quantify, but most studies state that around 15–20% have bilateral symptoms and as many as 60% may have radiological features of a minor asymptomatic slip.

1.27 ABC

A fracture haematoma aids fracture healing by sealing off the fracture site and providing a framework for the influx of inflammatory cells and fibroblasts. Factors such as FGF and PDGF, which are released by inflammatory cells, stimulate osteoprogenitor cells to differentiate into osteoblasts and osteoclasts. The histology of healing bone shows disorganised elements of bone formation and destruction (osteoblastic and osteoclastic activity) and has a similar picture to that in an osteosarcoma. It usually takes a minimum of 3 weeks for calcified tissue (callus) to be seen on X-ray in an adult. Reduced callus formation occurs when fracture movement is minimised, e.g. following internal fixation.

1.28 BCDE

Infection is an early complication of fractures, especially when open. Ideally, open fractures should be fixed within 4–6 hours of injury. All patients with open fractures should be given antibiotics. Volkmann's ischaemic contracture occurs following an arterial injury or compartment syndrome where muscle is replaced by inelastic fibrous tissue. This may leading to claw hand or toes. Tendon rupture is a well-recognised late complication of fractures. Extensor pollicis longus rupture occurs (6–12 weeks) after fracture of the lower radius, and the long head of biceps may rupture following a humeral neck fracture. Myositis ossificans is a form of heterotopic calcification occurring in soft tissue notably after dislocation of the elbow or a blow to the brachialis, deltoid or quadriceps. Treatment includes initial rest then gentle active movements. Occasionally excision of the bony mass is required. Algodystrophy (Sudek's atrophy) is characterised by a painful post-traumatic extremity. Late trophic changes are seen with features of patchy osteoporosis on X-ray.

1.29 ABDE

Non-union is caused by: unrecognised delayed union; wide distraction and separation of the fracture surfaces; and soft tissue interposition, excessive movement at the fracture site or poor local blood supply. Painless movement at the fracture site is diagnostic of non-union, as distinct from delayed union which is painful. Two types of non-union are described: hypertrophic (bulbous bone ends) and atrophic (no calcification at bone ends). Non-union is occasionally symptomless, needing no treatment. Functional bracing may induce union and electrical stimulation may promote osteogenesis. Bone grafts are required for atrophic non-union. Management includes functional bracing, electrical stimulation and internal or external fixation. Bone grafts are required for atrophic non-union.

1.30 BCE

Causes of delayed union include an inadequate blood supply, infection, incorrect immobilisation and intact fellow bone (such as the fibula in a tibial fracture). The fracture site is usually tender and the fracture remains visible with very little callus formation, periosteal reaction or sclerosis at the bone ends. Continued treatment is required and includes functional bracing, an excellent method of promoting bony union. A fracture should undergo internal fixation and bone grafting if union is delayed for more than 6 months and in the absence of any callus formation.

1.31 AC

Predisposing factors to recurrent dislocation include: generalised ligamentous laxity; underdevelopment of the lateral femoral condyle and flattening of the intercondylar groove; maldevelopment of the patella; valgus deformity of the knee; and a primary muscle defect. Recurrent dislocation of the patella is a known cause of osteoarthritis, and is more common in girls and often bilateral.

1.32 AB

There are four cardinal signs of osteoarthritis on an X-ray: asymmetrical joint space narrowing; sclerosis of subchondral bone; osteophytes at the joint margins; and bone cysts close to the joint surface. Symmetrical joint space narrowing and periarticular osteoporosis are features of rheumatoid arthritis.

1.33 BCDF

Paget's disease of bone is characterised by enlargement and thickening of the bone but the internal architecture is abnormal and the bone is unusually brittle. It affects men and women equally, most commonly from the age of 50 years. The most commonly affected sites are the pelvis and tibia. An elevated alkaline phosphatase indicates increased osteoblastic activity. Complications include nerve compression, fractures, osteoarthritis, osteosarcoma, high-output cardiac failure and hypercalcaemia. Treatment focuses on suppressing bone turnover and includes the use of calcitonin and bisphosphonates. Surgery may be required for pathological fractures and nerve entrapment states.

1.34 DE

Calcitonin acts to oppose parathyroid hormone, i.e. it causes increased renal excretion and reduces bone resorption. Vitamin D is produced in the skin by sunlight and ingested in the diet. It first undergoes 25-hydroxylation in the liver and then 1α-hydroxylation in the kidney to form the active 1,25-dihydroxycholecalciferol (1,25-DHCC). This last stage is under the control of PTH and phosphorus. A rise in PTH or a fall in serum phosphate increases 1,25-DHCC synthesis. Oestrogen increases calcium absorption and protects against the unopposed action of PTH.

1.35 AC

Bone or joints are affected in about 5% of patients with TB. Vertebral bodies and large synovial joints are the most commonly affected sites. Granulation tissue may extend across the joint and articular cartilage, thereby causing bone erosion and local osteoporosis. There is little or no periosteal reaction. Synovial fluid yields the diagnosis in only 10–20% of cases. A synovial biopsy is required to obtain specimens for culture (positive in over 80% of cases) and histology.

1.36 ADF

In club foot (talipes equinovarus) the foot is held in equinovarus, i.e. downwards and inwards. Boys are twice as likely to be affected as girls. The condition may be associated with spina bifida myelomeningocele. The objectives of treatment are to correct the deformity early and fully, and to hold the corrected position until the foot stops growing. The initial treatment is that of splintage, where the deformity is 'overcorrected'. Resistant cases will require surgery in the form of a tendon release and fixation.

1.37 AC

Osteomyelitis may occur after any operation on bone, but especially after implantation of foreign material, e.g. prostheses. The organisms may come from the theatre environment, patient, surgeon or indirectly from a distant focus. It may present early (within 3 months) or late. The organisms are usually a mixture of pathogenic bacteria (*Staphylococcus. aureus, Proteus* spp., *Pseudomonas* spp.). Predisposing factors include soft tissue damage, bone death, poor contact between implant and bone, loosening and corrosion of the implant. Elimination of any focus of infection, optimal operative sterility, prophylactic antibiotics, close fit and secure fixation of the implant will reduce the risk of postoperative osteomyelitis. MRI is not helpful in the early infection as it cannot distinguish between infection and normal postoperative changes. However, it may demonstrate collections of pus in late infections.

1.38 ABE

This is caused by compression and ischaemia of the median nerve within the carpal tunnel. Pain and paraesthesia characteristically occur at night in the distribution of the median nerve in the hand. It is associated with rheumatoid arthritis, pregnancy and hypothyroidism, and is more common around the time of the menopause. It is eight times more common in women. Froment's test is for ulnar nerve function, a positive Tinel's 'tapping' test involves gently tapping over the median nerve; a positive Tinel's sign occurs if paraesthesia occurs in the distribution of the median nerve, and this sign may be seen in carpal tunnel syndrome. Nerve conduction studies show a characteristic slowing of nerve conduction across the wrist.

1.39 EF

This is nodular thickening and contracture of the superficial palmar fascia. It is associated with thickening of the plantar aponeurosis and, in rare cases, fibrosis of the corpus cavernosum (Peyronie's disease). Dupuytren's contracture may be inherited as an autosomal dominant trait and is most common in people of European origin. It is associated with alcoholic cirrhosis, diabetes mellitus and phenytoin therapy, and usually affects the ring finger first. The digital nerve is displaced but not invaded. Operation is indicated if the deformity is a nuisance or rapidly progressing. Fasciectomy or excision of thickened fascia is the usual operation. Amputation is occasionally needed if there is severe contracture that the patient finds disabling.

1.40 BCD

Injury to the radial nerve may occur as it travels in the spiral groove of the humerus. It is common, but recovery is usual, especially in closed fractures. Fractures of the humerus heal readily and require neither perfect reduction nor immobilisation. The weight of the arm with an external cast is usually sufficient to bring the fragments into alignment. Spiral fractures unite in about 6 weeks, other varieties in 10–12 weeks. Delayed union may occur in transverse fractures. Child abuse must be considered in humeral shaft fractures.

1.41 CE

Perthes' disease is uncommon, with an incidence of about 1 in 10,000, and is particularly rare in the Afro-Caribbean population. This disease affects boys:girls 4:1. It presents between the ages of 4 and 8 years with a painful limp. The condition is due to avascular necrosis of the femoral head. The presentation coincides with the switch in blood supply of the femoral head from the femoral shaft vessels to ligamentum teres vessels. During this period the femoral head depends heavily on the lateral epiphyseal vessels which are vulnerable to damage. It is more common in Caucasian boys of social class V in underprivileged communities. Abduction is nearly always limited and internal rotation too is limited.

1.42 BE

These types of injuries either occur due to an indirect force, such as a fall on to the hand, or a direct blow to the forearm. In children the fracture is often incomplete with only minor angulation needed. Closed reduction is usually successful in children. In adults, unless the fragments are in close apposition, reduction is difficult and redisplacement in the cast is almost invariable, hence open reduction and internal fixation is favoured by most surgeons. Nerve injury due to the fracture is rare. There is good collateral circulation, thus injury to the radial or ulnar artery seldom presents any problem. Cross-union between the two bones prevents rotation.

1.43 ABCE

Internal fixation is often the most desirable form of treatment. The main indications for internal fixation are fractures that are unstable, unite slowly, pathological fractures, multiple fractures or where there may be nursing difficulties. Fixation of multiple fractures reduces the risk of general complications and late multiple-organ failure. If the bones have been fixed rigidly with the ends apart, the fracture may fail to unite. Iatrogenic infection is now the most common cause of chronic osteitis.

1.44 ACDEF

Pelvic fractures are commonly associated with bladder and urethral injuries. Damage to iliac arteries and veins can precipitate fatal hypovolaemic shock. Bladder injuries may be extra- or intraperitoneal, depending on the mechanism of injury and state of bladder filling at the time. Madura foot is due to mycetoma pedis, a chronic fungal infection. Open pelvic fractures carry a mortality of 50%. Fat embolism is a complication of both open and closed fractures.

1.45 AB

The roof of the popliteal fossa is formed by the fascia lata. Within the apex of the fossa the sciatic nerve divides into common peroneal and tibial branches (but may divide higher), the former lies either against or under the medial edge of the biceps femoris muscle, and the deepest structure is the popliteal artery. The sural nerve pierces the deep fascia halfway down the leg. The roof is pierced by the short saphenous vein.

1.46 BD

In the natal cleft, the sacral cornua are important surface markings for the sacral hiatus through which a needle is passed for epidural anaesthesia. Direct inguinal hernia protrude above and medial to the pubic tubercle. The external inguinal ring is palpable superolateral to the pubic tubercle. The femoral canal has the lacunar ligament as its medial wall. The ischial spine guides a needle to the pudendal canal for per vaginum pudendal nerve block. The transtubercular plane is an important landmark for lumbar puncture and transects the L5 vertebra (the supracristal plane, which passes through the L4 lumbar spine, can also be used).

1.47 ABCD

The scaphoid articulates with the radius, and since it transmits weight from the hand to the radial head it is commonly fractured during falls. When the fracture line severs the blood supply to the proximal fragment, avascular necrosis of the latter is a common complication. Tenderness in the anatomical 'snuffbox' is initially the only clinical sign of the fracture before radiological evidence of osteonecrosis develops (2 weeks later). The flexor retinaculum takes its origin from the tubercle of the scaphoid and ridge on the trapezium. The adductor pollicis muscle has an origin from the capitate, not the scaphoid; thus adduction of the thumb is unimpaired and pain-free after scaphoid fracture.

1.48 CDE

The dorsalis pedis artery lies between the extensor hallucis longus tendon medially, and the deep peroneal nerve lies laterally. The L5 dermatome lies over the medial half of the dorsum of the foot. The great saphenous vein is found anterior to the medial malleolus, and the lower limb of the extensor retinaculum passes under the medial longitudinal arch and blends with the plantar aponeurosis.

1.49 ABD

Sympathetic grey rami connect with all spinal nerve roots. The nervi erigentes originate from S2, 3 and often 4. The lumbosacral trunk (L4/5) passes anterior to the alar of the sacrum, under cover of the common iliac vessels, and joins the S1 ventral ramus above the piriformis muscle. The adductor muscles are supplied by L2–4 roots of the lumbar plexus. They develop by medial migration from the flexor (hamstring) compartment, and are therefore supplied by anterior divisions.

1.50 B

The thoracodorsal nerve is vulnerable in axillary surgery because of its unprotected prominence on the posterior wall. The whole of the serratus anterior muscle (8 costal digitations: 1 and 2 into the superior angle; 3 and 4 whole vertebral border; lower 4 inferior angle) is used to protract the scapula, whilst the bulky insertion into the lower angle of the scapula aids the trapezius muscle in rotation. The long thoracic nerve (of Bell), which is protected underneath the fascia covering the serratus anterior muscle, innervates the muscle, originating from the C5–7 roots.

1.51 All false

Flexion and extension take place between lumbar vertebrae, but the articular facets limit rotation. The left crus of the diaphragm is attached to the first two lumbar vertebrae. The iliolumbar ligament attaches to the lateral process of the L5 vertebra. The central canal, at the level of the L3 vertebra, contains the cauda equina. The iliolumbar branch of the posterior division of the internal iliac artery supplies the L5 vertebra. Only paired segmental lumbar branches of the abdominal aorta supply L1–4 vertebrae.

1.52 BC

The antecubital fossa contains the posterior interosseous branch of the radial nerve (which leaves the fossa between the two heads of the supinator muscle) and the brachial artery (which lies lateral to the median nerve against the tendon of the biceps muscle). The brachial artery bifurcates within the fossa into radial and ulnar arteries. Part of the roof is formed by the bicipital aponeurosis, which separates the superficial median cubital vein from the contents of the fossa. The brachioradialis brachialis muscle and the medial edge of the supinator muscle form the floor.

1.53 AE

The carpal tunnel contains the median nerve, as well as the tendons of the flexor carpi radialis, flexor pollicis longus, and flexor digitorum alis superficialis and flexor digitorum profundus brevis tendons. The ulnar artery and nerve, and the flexor carpi ulnaris tendon, lie outside the tunnel. The flexor digitorum brevis is found in the foot.

1.54 ADE

The superficial epigastric and superficial external pudendal arteries pass through the saphenous opening (the superficial circumflex and deep external pudendal arteries pierce the fascia lata). The femoral artery separates the femoral nerve (laterally) from the femoral vein (medially). The profunda femoris artery is a lateral branch of the femoral artery. The deep inguinal nodes lie medial to the femoral vein. The femoral sheath encloses the femoral vessels for up to 3 cm beyond the inguinal ligament, where the sheath terminates by fusing with the adventitia of both vessels.

1.55 AD

Avascular necrosis occurs following an interruption of the arterial blood supply to a bone or following intra- or extraosseus venous insufficiency. Susceptible bones include the femoral and humeral heads, femoral condyles, capitum (when avulsed), proximal pole of the scaphoid, lunate and talus. The blood supply to the femoral head arises from the joint capsule. The femoral head is susceptible after an intracapsular (subcapital) but not an extracapsular (intertrochanteric) fracture.

1.56 D

Compartment syndrome results from an increased pressure within a closed compartment; thus with a grade 3b open fracture where there is gross disruption of the soft tissues, a compartment syndrome is rare. The syndrome is associated with pain on stretching the muscles in the involved compartment (i.e. extension or dorsiflexion) and is diagnosed when the pressure is 30 mmHg – hence peripheral pulses are unaffected.

1.57 AB

The patellar reflex is mediated by the femoral nerve formed from the posterior divisions of the L2–4 anterior spinal rami, and is thus lost after femoral nerve and L2–4 dorsal root damage. T12 cord lesions result in an upper motor neurone lesion with exaggerated reflexes. Dorsal column lesions only affect central sensory processing since collaterals subserving spinal reflexes are preserved.

1.58 CDE

Kanavel's cardinal signs of suppurative tenosynovitis of the flexor tendons are: fingers held in slight flexion; pain on passive movement; fusiform swelling; and tenderness along the flexor sheath extending into the palm. The patient is not usually systemically unwell.

1.59 Knee injuries

1. B Medial collateral ligament injury
2. D Patella fracture
3. F Posterior cruciate ligament tear
4. E Anterior cruciate ligament tear
5. A Medial meniscus tear

Tenderness above (or below) the joint line with laxity when a valgus or varus strain is applied to the knee is associated with injury to the medial or lateral collateral ligaments. Symptoms of instability are common and swelling may either be within or around the joint (depending on the degree of damage to the ligament). Tenderness over the joint line itself following injury is most suggestive of a meniscal injury. With a displaced bucket-handle tear, the knee may not extend (or indeed flex) fully. Symptoms may include pain, recurrent giving way and locking with clicking.

A hyperextension injury to the knee when associated with a 'pop' may represent injury to the ACL. As this is an intra-articular injury, swelling is often immediate and due to bleeding (haemarthrosis). Laxity may not always be obvious initially unless the patient is anaesthetised. Later, symptoms such as giving way and pain become increasingly troublesome.

The posterior cruciate ligament prevents the femur from sliding forwards off the tibial plateau, and in the weight-bearing flexed knee it is the only stabilising factor for the femur. Thus, going downstairs is often troublesome for people with deficiency of the posterior cruciate ligament. This ligament is quite frequently damaged with dashboard injuries such as that described in scenario 3. Diagnosis of knee injury may be delayed due to the overriding symptoms from the associated hip injury.

If the extensor mechanism contracts against resistance – e.g. when the foot is caught in a hole or on an uneven paving stone – it is likely to fail. In the young patient the patellar tendon ruptures, in the older patient the quadriceps tendon fails. In between – the patella may fracture (usually transverse with displacement). A direct blow to the front of the knee is likely to lead to a stellate fracture. If the extensor mechanism is damaged, the patient may be unable to lift their leg and walking is difficult. As the joint has been 'ruptured' the swelling is usually not a discrete effusion.

1.60 Shoulder pain
1. E Avascular necrosis
2. D Bone cyst
3. C Osteosarcoma
4. B Osteomyelitis

Avascular necrosis is quite common following long-term steroid therapy (usually >2 years). In its early stages there may be no X-ray features but MRI changes are diagnostic.

Bone cysts usually occur in the metaphyses of long bones. They are lytic lesions with well-defined sclerotic margins.

Osteosarcomas also affect the metaphyses of long bones and present in the 2nd and 3rd decades of life. They may have a mixed lytic and sclerotic appearance with a poorly defined margin.

Osteomyelitis often affects the metaphyseal region of long bones and there may be a history of a preceding upper respiratory tract infection. X-ray changes may be minimal if the condition has been picked up in the early stages but may mimic an osteosarcoma.

Acute calcific tendonitis is most common in young adults and calcific deposits in the soft tissues may be seen on X-ray. The shoulder is acutely painful and movement of the joint may be impossible. The differential diagnosis would include a septic arthritis.

1.61 B

The head of the radius articulates with the lateral two carpal bones, and it is thus the radius and not the ulna that usually fractures after a fall on the outstretched hand. Isolated ulnar fractures usually occur after a direct blow. Since the ulna does not articulate at the wrist, movement at the wrist is unimpaired. Similarly, movements of the little finger, mediated by the superficial and deep flexors and extensors, are unaffected as the lower end of the ulna does not give attachment to these muscles. Pronation is, however, impaired because of pain resulting either from involvement of the inferior radioulnar joint or movement of the fracture site across the attachment of the pronator quadratus muscle.

1.62 ACD

The musculocutaneous nerve (C5, C6) is a branch of the lateral cord of the brachial plexus and supplies the biceps. Each C5 and C6 spinal nerve is formed from dorsal (sensory) and ventral (motor) roots, mediating the afferent and efferent reflex arcs, respectively. Each spinal nerve divides into a dorsal and ventral ramus. The C5/6 ventral rami form the upper trunk of the brachial plexus. The lateral cord is formed from anterior divisions of the upper (C5/6) and middle (C7) trunks. Thus, neither the medial cord nor the middle trunk mediates the reflex.

1.63 Femoral fractures

1. E Austin–Moore hemiarthroplasty
2. C Cannulated screw fixation
3. B Sliding compression screw with 2-hole plate
4. G Reconstruction femoral nail

Undisplaced and impacted fractures in patients of all ages should be treated by internal fixation. Preservation of the femoral head is the aim if possible.

In the young patient with minimal displacement, cannulated screws would be used.

In patients over the age of 65 years, the chance of non-union and avascular necrosis is high, thus a hemiarthroplasty is performed.

Concomitant femoral shaft and neck fractures may be managed with a reconstruction nail or a sliding compression screw with a long plate. Both these implants have a screw that enters the femoral head, fixing the neck of femur in place.

A standard intramedullary femoral nail has a proximal locking screw that runs from the greater to lesser trochanters and would therefore not treat a femoral neck fracture.

1.64 All true

All muscles that insert into the extensor expansion extend the fingers at the interphalangeal joints. The lumbrical and interosseous muscles also flex the first metacarpophalangeal joints. The radial nerve is a branch of the posterior cord of the brachial plexus and innervates the long extensor muscles. The ulnar nerve supplies the two ulnar lumbrical muscles and all the interosseous muscles. The two radial lumbrical muscles are supplied by the palmar digital branches of the median nerve.

1.65 ADE

Avascular necrosis of bone is a recognised complication of sickle-cell disease, decompression sickness and Gaucher's disease (a familial disorder common in Ashkenazi Jews). It may also be due to irradiation and drugs (particularly corticosteroids, alcohol and immunosuppressants). Although haemophilia A and B are associated with arthritis, they are not a recognised cause of avascular necrosis. Hunter's disease is a glycogen storage disorder but is not associated with avascular necrosis.

1.66 Nerve injury in the arm

1. F Posterior interosseous nerve and superficial radial nerve injury in the forearm

2. C Ulnar nerve injury at the elbow

The radial nerve divides into the posterior interosseous nerve (motor) and superficial radial nerve (sensory) in the cubital fossa. Mid-forearm injuries of the radial nerve will have preserved wrist extension, as the innervation to the extensor carpi radialis longus muscle is preserved via a proximal branch of the posterior interosseous nerve before it pierces the supinator muscle. Thus, although there is weakness of wrist extension, wrist drop is avoided. Branches to the triceps arise in the axillas, proximal to the spiral groove.

Ulnar nerve injury at the wrist causes paralysis of the intrinsic muscles of hand, with wasting of the interossei and hypothenar muscles.

1.67 BE

The superficial palmar arch is incomplete over the thenar eminence. The radial artery passes over the dorsum of the wrist. The flexor digitorum superficialis tendons lie in the carpal tunnel medial to the median nerve and thenar eminence. All these structures therefore escape damage from a deep laceration into the thenar eminence. However, the recurrent branch of the median nerve and the adductor pollicis muscle would be involved, and thus movements of the thumb would be restricted.

1.68 ABCD

Abduction of the arms is initiated by the supraspinatus muscle over the first 15°, and then continues to hold the head of the humerus against the glenoid cavity. The deltoid muscle then takes over and, at about 90°, the arm is laterally rotated mainly by the infraspinatus muscle (both the supraspinatus and infraspinatus muscles stabilise the shoulder joint by tightening the rotator cuff). The scapula is then rotated by the combined actions of the trapezius and the inferior fibres of the serratus anterior muscles. The teres major muscle is a medial rotator and not part of the rotator cuff.

1.69 ACD

Nerve root involvement is suggested by pain radiating below the knee. It is worse when the nerve is stretched, as with the sciatic stretch test, or when intra-abdominal pressure is raised, as with straining at stool, coughing or sneezing. Urinary retention is a worrying sign but is not infrequently secondary to pain, analgesic medication and bedrest. Before this can be assumed, a full neurological examination must be performed; if there are concerns regarding a cauda equina syndrome then further investigations must be carried out. An absent ankle jerk implies some nerve root damage, but on its own does not demand surgical intervention.

1.70 BCD

The four classic signs are loss of joint space, bony sclerosis and cyst formation in the weight-bearing areas of the joint, and osteophyte formation at the joint margins. Periarticular erosions are classically found in rheumatoid arthritis.

1.71 CE

Fat embolism is most common in patients with multiple closed fractures. It may also occur following burns and cardiac surgery. The clinical features of fat embolism include dyspnoea, mental confusion, restlessness and petechiae in the conjunctival folds and on the chest. There is no specific test for fat embolism but a fairly constant finding is hypoxaemia. Treatment is supportive, involving ventilation as required.

1.72 BDE

The principles of management of a compound fracture include a full assessment of the patient and thus the ABCs of trauma must be included. The assessment against the GCS is also appropriate. Management should also include parenteral antibiotics, antiseptic dressing, analgesia, antitetanus treatment and alignment of the limb with immobilisation. (The 5As.) A plaster cast will not immobilise a proximal femoral fracture – traction would be more appropriate.

1.73 Back pain
1. D **Spondylolysis**
2. E **Discitis**
3. B **Scheuermann's disease**
4. C **TB of the spine**
5. F **Facet joint arthritis**

Spondylolysis is a defect in the pars interarticularis and is often associated with a slip (spondylolisthesis). The defect may arise as a stress fracture, which is associated with significant pain, and is particularly common in young aggressive fast bowlers.

Discitis may be secondary to a haematogenous infection, but it is more commonly due to direct inoculation of organisms following an invasive procedure on a disc. In this case it could have been due to prolapse of retained disc material, but the inflammatory markers here are higher than one would normally expect to see in the postoperative period. Both scoliosis and kyphosis may be classed as curvatures of the spine. The kyphosis associated with Scheuermann's disease is slightly more common in boys and often associated with aching pain, whilst idiopathic scoliosis is more common in girls who are usually pain-free.

In areas where TB is still widespread, infection of the spine is quite common. A history of longstanding back pain with signs of chronic ill health should raise the possibility of this diagnosis.

Unaccustomed exercise is likely to precipitate symptoms from arthritic joints, and the back is no exception. A prolapsed disc is unlikely at 60 years of age and facet joint pain may radiate as far as the knee.

1.74 ABDE

Open fractures are more appropriately treated by external fixation because of the increased risk of infection, but if a closed fracture is converted to an open fracture in order to deal with a soft tissue or vascular injury then internal fixation is advised. Similarly, failure to obtain or maintain a satisfactory reduction of a fracture by closed means dictates that an open reduction be considered. This is followed by internal fixation if appropriate. Pathological fractures are likely to heal slowly (if at all) and thus internal fixation methods allow prompt mobilisation.

1.75 BDE

The piriformis muscle lies partly within the pelvis and emerges through the greater sciatic foramen to enter the gluteal region. The structures passing or emerging from the upper border of the piriformis muscle include the superior gluteal nerve and vessels. Below the lower border of the piriformis emerge the inferior gluteal nerve and muscles, pudendal nerve and vessels, the nerve to obturator internus and the sciatic nerve.

1.76 ACEF

The tibial nerve is the large terminal branch of the sciatic nerve. It runs through the popliteal fossa, at first lying on the lateral side, then crossing medial to the popliteal artery. It leaves the fossa by passing deep to the gastrocnemius and soleus. The tibial nerve supplies the knee joint, popliteus, the posterior compartment muscles of the leg and the foot.

1.77 Bone disease

1. **B Avascular necrosis**
2. **F Osteosarcoma**
3. **C Rickets**
4. **A Paget's disease**
5. **G Osteochondroma**

Steroids are an important cause of avascular necrosis, which is itself painful. Bow-legs in a 2-year-old child may be normal, but rickets must be considered in the presence of expanded metaphyses, rickety rosary, failure to thrive, general lassitude and muscle weakness.

In the adult, increasing bony deformity with or without pain is often associated with Paget's disease. Paget's disease may affect the skull, giving rise to conductive deafness. Paget's disease may also give rise to spinal stenosis, osteoarthritis, pathological fractures and sarcomatous changes (chondrosarcoma, osteosarcoma, fibrosarcoma).

Osteosarcomas generally present in the second and third decades with swelling, pain, tenderness and loss of function. It is classic for a patient to present with a history of trauma, although it is completely unrelated to the pathology.

Osteochondromas occur around the same areas but usually produce much more discrete swellings and should stop increasing in size by the time of skeletal maturity. The patient in Scenario 5 has diaphyseal aclasis, a condition of multiple osteochondromas. Osteochondromas are cartilage-capped and metaphyseal in location. They are benign tumours affecting the 10–12-year age group, with a male predominance.

1.78 BCDE

Acute osteomyelitis is most often found in children. In adults it is associated with immunosuppression and diabetes. The organism is most commonly *Staphylococcus aureus.* Others include *Streptococcus pyogenes* and *S. pneumoniae.* In children <4 years, *Haemophilus influenzae* is fairly common. Patients with sickle-cell are more prone to salmonella infection. Organisms settle in the metaphysis, most often at the proximal end of the femur. In adults, the thoracolumbar spine is the most common site for haematogenous infection. X-ray changes (lytic or sclerotic changes, periosteal reaction) usually take 10 days to 2 weeks to become apparent. The first X-ray change seen is that of soft tissue swelling.

ANSWERS – CHAPTER 2: VASCULAR

2.1 ABEF

The IVC commences opposite the L5 vertebra formed by the confluence of the right and left common iliac veins. It runs on the right of the aorta upwards towards the diaphragm, it extends to the central tendinous diaphragm at the level of the body of the T8 vertebra. The IVC lies posterior to the bare area and caudate lobe of the liver. Due to its compound embryological origin, the tributaries are not identical to the branches of the abdominal aorta. On the right side, the testicular vein drains into the inferior vena cava; but on the left, the testicular vein drains into the left renal vein.

2.2 DE

The middle meningeal artery divides from the maxillary branch of the external carotid, entering the cranium through the foramen spinosum. It is the largest artery that supplies the dura. While the maxillary artery does give off branches in the pterygopalatine fossa region, the middle meningeal artery comes off more proximally deep to the ramus of the mandible.

2.3 Anatomy of the pelvic vasculature

1. F Lateral sacral veins
2. B Superior vesical artery
3. E Inferior vesical artery
4. D Superior rectal vein

The lateral sacral veins directly communicate with the vertebral venous plexus by valveless tributaries, and are thus a pathway for metastases from pelvic tumours to pass to the vertebrae.

The superior vesical artery is the persistent patent proximal part of the fetal umbilical artery. The distal part becomes obliterated to form the medial umbilical ligament.

The inferior vesical artery supplies the prostate gland.

The superior rectal vein drains into the inferior mesenteric vein and thus into the portal system.

2.4 AB

As soon as the aorta passes below the aortic hiatus, it gives off the coeliac plexus (T12). The plexus has three direct branches: left gastric, hepatic and splenic (mnemonic: **l**eft **h**and **s**ide). The right gastric and gastroduodenal arteries are branches of the hepatic artery. The superior pancreatico-duodenal artery is a branch of the gastroduodenal artery.

2.5 EF

The right common carotid artery branches off the brachiocephalic artery. It bifurcates at the level of the upper border of the lamina of the thyroid cartilage. It lies posterior to the lobes of the thyroid gland and anterior to both the cervical sympathetic chain and the phrenic nerve on the scalenus anterior muscle, the latter is separated from the artery by prevertebral fascia.

2.6 ACDE

The basilic vein is a continuation of the ulnar stem of the dorsal venous arch in the hand. It lies medial to the biceps tendon in the cubital fossa and is medial to the medial cutaneous nerve of the forearm in the arm. The basilic vein ascends in the superficial fascia on the medial side of the biceps. It then pierces the deep fascia in the middle of the upper arm, is joined by the venae comitantes of the brachial artery, and becomes the axillary vein at the lower border of the teres major muscle.

2.7 ACDE

The popliteal artery divides into the anterior and posterior tibial arteries at the lower border of the popliteus muscle, anterior to the fibrous arch of the soleus muscle. The peroneal artery is the first branch of the posterior tibial artery. At the ankle joint, the posterior tibial artery passes deep to the flexor retinaculum.

2.8 Aortic bypass grafting

1. A Aortobifemoral bypass
2. B Axillobifemoral bypass
3. A Aortobifemoral bypass

An aortobifemoral bypass graft has the highest patency rate of any bypass procedures to the femoral vessels.
An axillobifemoral bypass graft should only be considered in the very high risk surgical patient who has critical ischaemia. It should not be performed in patients with claudication.

2.9 Lower limb ischaemia
1. B Percutaneous balloon angioplasty
2. C Femorodistal bypass
3. E Tissue plasminogen activator (TPA) infusion (intra-arterial)
4. G Lifestyle changes only
5. F Fasciotomy

Percutaneous balloon angioplasty is particularly suitable for localised stenoses and short occlusions. Lesions in the larger proximal vessels (above knee) are technically easier to treat, with fewer complications and better long-term results.

Femorodistal bypass using an autogenous vein graft is the treatment of choice in the second patient. Absence of contrast in the posterior tibial, anterior tibial and common peroneal arteries on angiography films must not be accepted as evidence of their occlusion.

Intra-arterial thrombolysis with TPA is the treatment of choice in the third patient in view of the short history (4 hours), angiographic findings and absence of neurological deficit.

The initial treatment of intermittent claudication is correction of risk factors, such as diabetes, hypertension, smoking and exercise. Younger, non-smokers should have a thrombotic screen performed on presentation.

Critical ischaemia is defined by rest pain of at least 2 weeks' duration that requires regular adequate analgesia, or ulceration or gangrene of the foot or toes with an ankle pressure of <50 mmHg or a toe pressure of <30 mmHg.

The fifth patient has compartment syndrome. Urgent fasciotomy is indicated in order to save his right leg.

2.10 ACF

The aorta enters the abdomen under the median arcuate ligament at T12 and divides into the common iliac arteries at L4 (intercristal plane). The cisterna chyli lies under cover of the right crus of the diaphragm, with the azygous vein on the right and the aorta to the left. In its course through the abdomen, the aorta gives off the 3 single ventral gut arteries (coeliac, superior and inferior mesenteric) and passes under the left renal vein. Unless the patient is obese, abdominal aortic pulsations are normally palpable.

2.11 ABCE

The surface marking of the femoral artery is the mid-inguinal point that lies just medial to the position of the deep inguinal ring, which is at the midpoint of the inguinal ligament. The perforating branches of the profunda femoris artery supply the hamstrings. Branches of the circumflex femoral arteries contribute to the trochanteric anastomosis which feed the femoral head via their subretinacular branches. The femoral artery is subcutaneous in the femoral triangle, separated from skin by the fascia lata.

2.12 Lower limb venous disease

1. A Elevation, rest, NSAIDs and antibiotics
2. C IV heparin
3. B Emergency surgery

The woman with thrombosed varicose veins and cellulitis should be treated with elevation, rest, NSAIDs and antibiotics.
One should also suspect a deep vein thrombosis in a patient with a swollen and tender leg postoperatively. It is best to perform some imaging (duplex Doppler study) before commencing treatment for this second scenario.
A patient with venous insufficiency with profuse bleeding from an ulcer should have emergency surgery to stop the bleeding.

2.13 BCE

The portal vein is formed by the confluence of the superior mesenteric vein (lying to the right of the artery) and the splenic vein behind the neck of the pancreas. It is about 5 cm long. The terminals of the portal vein and the hepatic artery form, with the hepatic ductules, the triads of the liver in the corners of the hexagonal lobules. The central veins drain into the hepatic veins.

2.14 Carotid artery disease

1. B Carotid Doppler
2. A CT scan

30% of carotid bruits heard on auscultation are not due to carotid stenosis. The initial investigation that should be performed is a Doppler ultrasound scan in patient 1. This may be followed by digital subtraction angiography or MRA, but many centres will rely on colour duplex Doppler alone if performed by an experienced operator.
In cases where a persistent neurological deficit has occurred then a CT scan must be carried out initially to exclude a space-occupying lesion.

2.15 AC

When ligating the inferior thyroid arteries, the recurrent laryngeal nerves are vulnerable. When ligating the superior thyroid arteries, the external laryngeal nerves running alongside may be damaged. The internal laryngeal nerves pass above and behind the root of the superior thyroid arteries and are thus usually outside the operative field. The phrenic nerves are protected as they lie behind the prevertebral fascia. Both transverse cervical nerves run in the subcutaneous fascia. Horizontal skin-crease thyroidectomy incisions run parallel with their course and thus most branches of these cutaneous nerves are spared.

2.16 ABDE

The brachial artery begins at the lower border of the teres major terminating opposite the neck of the radius by branching into the radial and ulnar arteries. Its pulse can be palpated as it descends the arm overlapped by the medial border of the biceps muscle. The median nerve crosses over it (from lateral to medial) roughly before the artery's midpoint. Initially in the upper arm, the ulnar nerve travels alongside lying posteriorly, but more distally, it leaves the artery after piercing the medial intermuscular septum. The artery is surrounded by venae comitantes, reinforced by the basilic vein. In the cubital fossa, the artery is overlain by the bicipital aponeurosis but it passes over the biceps tendon.

2.17 Investigation of carotid artery disease

1. A Duplex Doppler ultrasound of carotid arteries
2. C CT scan of head
3. E Transcranial Doppler ultrasound

Duplex Doppler ultrasound of the carotid arteries is the initial investigation of choice for carotid stenosis. It is the quickest and safest investigation for amaurosis fugax. Carotid angiography or MRA may be used subsequently to confirm the duplex findings.

The 28-year-old with the dense stroke is most likely to have had an intracranial bleed necessitating a CT of the brain.

Transcranial Doppler measures the flow in the middle cerebral artery and is thus useful in the intraoperative monitoring and investigation of postendarterectomy neurological episodes. Duplex Doppler would also demonstrate patency of the carotid artery following endarterectomy. Near-infrared spectroscopy measures intracerebral blood flow but is not currently used for intraoperative monitoring.

2.18 ABD

The blood supply to the breast is mainly from the lateral thoracic artery. The internal thoracic artery, perforating intercostal arteries and the pectoral branches of the thoracoacromial artery also contribute. Venous return simply follows the arteries mentioned above. The nipple is a reliable marker for the T4 dermatome. In the breast 75% of the lymph drains through the axillary nodes. The retromammary space overlies the pectoralis major muscle.

2.19 AC

The thoracic duct begins below the diaphragm as the cysterna chyli and then ascends through the aortic opening in the diaphragm, to the right of the descending aorta. It passes behind the oesophagus and then to the left of the oesophagus at the level of T5. It then runs upwards on the left side of the oesophagus into the neck. Here it crosses the subclavian artery to enter the left brachiocephalic vein. At the root of the neck, the thoracic duct receives the left jugular, subclavian and bronchomediastinal lymph trunks, although they may occasionally drain directly into the adjacent large vessels. The thoracic duct thus conveys all the lymph from the lower limbs, pelvic cavity, abdominal cavity, left side of the thorax, head and neck and the left arm

2.20 B

Lymphoedema usually occurs following radiotherapy, fibrosis or infection and is usually painless. Subclinical lymphoedema may occur after venous thrombosis. Lymphangiography and technetium-99m colloid scans reveal lymphatic clearance and are commonly used investigations. 90% of all patients with primary or secondary lymphoedema respond readily to active conservative treatment. Diuretics are inadvisable.

2.21 ACD

The term 'lymphoedema' should be confined to describing oedema in patients in whom a lymphatic abnormality has been confirmed. Lymphoedema predominantly affects the legs (80%). The most common cause of unilateral ankle oedema is long-standing venous disease. 90% of patients respond to active conservative treatment consisting of pneumatic compression devices and elastic stockings. Cellulitis is more common in lymphoedema and if present should be aggressively treated with systemic antibiotics. Surgery is appropriate only in a few patients and consists of: debulking operations, or lymphatic bypass (mesenteric bridge procedure and lymphovenous anastomosis). The debulking operations remove excess subcutaneous tissue to improve lymphatic drainage in the skin.

2.22 CEF

The function of lymphatic vessels is to return the plasma capillary filtrate to the circulation. This task is achieved by increased tissue pressure, facilitated by intermittent skeletal muscle activity, contractions of lymphatic vessels and an extensive system of one-way valves. Lymphoedema is an accumulation of tissue fluid as a result of a fault in the lymphatic system – very often, many patients are diagnosed as having lymphoedema when the oedema is due to another cause. Lymphoedema can occur as a result of lymphatic obstruction secondary to infiltration of lymph nodes, frequently deep in the pelvis.

2.23 ABCD

Surgery is difficult, but there is a greater risk of complications with re-do surgery. Investigation is therefore important. Groin recurrences are most common. The long saphenous vein must be disconnected, flush with the femoral vein, and all the tributaries near their termination should be ligated and divided to prevent recurrences. Stripping of the long saphenous vein to the knee is associated with a lower recurrence rate.
Duplex ultrasound is valuable in determining the presence of retrograde flow in incompetent and/or communicating veins. It should therefore be part of the investigation of patients with varicose veins.

2.24 CD

The groin incision is over the saphenofemoral junction, which is medial to the femoral artery. An oblique, groin-crease incision is commonly used for primary varicose vein surgery. A longitudinal incision is popular for re-do varicose vein surgery. The named venous tributaries are the superficial and deep external pudendal, the superficial circumflex iliac and the superficial inferior epigastric. These tributaries should be ligated to reduce the risk of recurrence. The long saphenous vein is stripped to the knee to reduce recurrence. Stripping to the ankle does not afford any further benefit and is associated with increased morbidity, especially nerve injury.

2.25 DE

The abdominal aorta is the most frequent site of aneurysm formation and is found in 2% of all postmortems. Dilatation usually begins below the renal arteries and extends variably to the iliac veins. Only 2% of abdominal aortic aneurysms (AAA) extend above the renal arteries. The incidence of AAA appears greater in the elderly (above 60 years), males and hypertensives who smoke.

Most patients with a 6-cm aneurysm should be offered surgical repair, providing they are medically fit and can be expected to survive the operation. The latest study has demonstrated that small aneurysms, i.e. <5 cm, may be treated conservatively with regular surveillance.

Most aneurysms contain a thin rim of calcification in their walls, but overlying gas, colonic material or X-ray scatter may sometimes make them hard to see on AXR.

2.26 Lymph nodes

1. A Para-aortic
2. D External iliac
3. B Superficial inguinal
4. A Para-aortic

Lymphatics from the testicles run with the arteries and drain into the aortic nodes. Lymphatic spread of tumour from the cervix occurs in 40% of women, with preferential spread to the external iliac, internal iliac and obturator nodes. Drainage from the anal canal is to the internal iliac nodes from the upper part, and to the superficial inguinal nodes from the lower part. Lymphatic vessels from the rectum pass directly to the aortic nodes.

2.27 AB

The aorta enters the abdomen through the aortic hiatus of the diaphragm between the crura at the T12 level. The left lumbar veins pass behind it; anteriorly the aorta is related to the pancreas, which separates it from the stomach, the third part of the duodenum and colic of the small intestine. The aorta ends by dividing at the L4 level. Branches of the abdominal aorta are as follows:

3 unpaired anterior branches:

1. coeliac trunk
2. superior mesenteric artery (SMA)
3. inferior mesenteric artery (IMA)

3 lateral paired visceral branches:
1. adrenal
2. renal
3. gonadal

5 lateral paired parietal branches:
1. inferior phrenic
2. four pairs of lumbar arteries

Terminal branches:
1. common iliac arteries
2. median sacral artery

The lumbar sympathetic trunk lies against the lumbar vertebral bodies. The left sympathetic trunk is overlapped by the abdominal aorta and the right sympathetic trunk by the inferior vena cava.

2.28 ABCD

Carotid endarterectomy has a mortality of 1–2% in experienced hands with a stroke risk of 1–2%, but these figures are doubled if less-experienced surgeons operate. Complications of a carotid endarterectomy include damage to the VIIth, IXth, Xth and XIIth cranial nerves, perioperative or postoperative stroke, MI and wound infection. Patients should be on long-term aspirin therapy postoperatively.

2.29 ABCD

The vagus nerve travels in the carotid sheath in the neck. The sympathetic trunk lies alongside the cervical vertebrae, immediately behind the carotid artery, and has three cervical ganglion (superior, middle and inferior). During a left carotid endarterectomy (CEA), the thoracic duct may be seen. Pleural membranes are usually a little deeper and lateral to the site of CEA. The hypoglossal nerve passes forwards to supply the tongue and has to be protected, whilst the facial vein has to be ligated and divided to mobilise the internal jugular vein.

2.30 Types of ulceration
1. C Marjolin's ulcer
2. B Cushing's ulcer
3. A Curling's ulcer
4. E Pyoderma gangrenosum

Marjolin's ulcers are squamous-cell carcinomas that develop in long-standing chronic venous ulcers. Gastroduodenal stress ulcers follow major trauma or sepsis. The pathophysiology is unclear, but is thought to relate to relative mucosal ischaemia, lack of oral alimentation and altered gastric mucous-barrier function. Specific forms of gastroduodenal stress ulceration include: Cushing's ulcer, which follows severe head injury; and Curling's ulcer, which follows major burns. Pyoderma gangrenosum occurs in inflammatory bowel disease, and is more common in ulcerative colitis than Crohn's disease.

2.31 ADE

The Brodie–Trendelenburg test is the emptying of the leg veins by elevation, application of a tourniquet, lowering of the leg and release of the tourniquet. If the veins fill on release of the tourniquet then the incompetence must lie above the level of the tourniquet.

Saphenofemoral incompetence can be treated by ligation of the long saphenous vein at the saphenofemoral junction – this is the Trendelenburg procedure.

2.32 AB

The cephalic vein arises from the radial side of the dorsal venous arch of the hand and runs up the radial border of the forearm. It gives off a branch (the median cubital vein) in the cubital fossa and runs up the arm, lateral to the biceps. It lies anterior and lateral to the biceps tendon but never medial. The cephalic vein drains into the axillary vein. The axillary vein forms at the lower border of the teres minor where the basilic vein joins the venae comitantes of the brachial artery. It does contain valves.

2.33 ABCDE

The mortality rate for below-knee amputation is 10% and that of above-knee amputation 20–40%. This reflects the high incidence of severe cardiovascular disease in these patients. At least 8 cm of tibia is required to fit a below-knee prosthesis, but 15 cm is desirable and the anterior border should be bevelled to remove the sharp edge of the tibial crest. Nerves are best cut cleanly under tension with a blade to reduce the incidence of neuroma formation. Insertion of an epidural catheter into the tibial nerve sheath with infusion of local anaesthetic may aid postoperative analgesia. An epidural placed 48 hours before amputation is also reported to reduce the incidence of phantom limb pain.

2.34 A

Autologous saphenous vein is the conduit of choice for lower limb arterial reconstruction, achieving primary patency rates of up to 90% at 1 year. In its absence, a good-quality cephalic or basilic vein is a viable alternative. There is no convincing evidence from randomised trials that the patency rates differ between in-situ and reversed saphenous vein, although single series may claim that one or other is superior. Expanded PTFE grafts are a useful conduit when no suitable vein is available. The patency rates for PTFE tend to be worse than those for vein. Endothelialisation of the proximal and distal ends of the graft occurs, but a full length of endothelium cannot be supported by this prosthetic material. Untreated human umbilical vein is antigenic, but processed grafts are made by tanning with glutaraldehyde to render them non-antigenic. They are covered with a Dacron mesh to reduce the incidence of aneurysmal dilatation and provide external support.

2.35 ABC

The arch of the aorta commences from the manubriosternal joint and passes backwards over the left bronchus to reach the body of T4 vertebra just to the left of the midline. The arch is crossed on its left side by the phrenic and vagus nerves as they pass downwards in front of and behind the lung root, respectively. The left vertebral artery and the right internal mammary artery come off the left and right subclavian arteries, respectively.

2.36 CE

Nerve conduction disappears after about 30 minutes of complete ischaemia. Permanent muscle injury ensues a few hours later if circulation is not restored. In established ischaemia, there is a risk of reperfusion injury where toxins are liberated into the blood and can cause cardiac arrest or renal failure. Compartment syndrome is a well-known sequence of limb ischaemia and is best prevented by performing fasciotomies.

2.37 Vascular tumours
1. C Chemodectoma
2. B Angiosarcoma
3. A Kaposi's sarcoma
4. D Glomus jugulare tumour

Chemodectomas originate from paraganglionic cells at the carotid bifurcation. If untreated, 5% metastasise within 10 years.

Angiosarcomas usually develop in the extremities. Although they are radiosensitive and respond to chemotherapy, radical amputation is still advised.

A Kaposi's sarcoma is a haemangiosarcoma, treated with a combination of chemo- and radiotherapy.

A glomus jugulare tumour arises at the jugular bulb. Excision is associated with palsies of the Xth, XIth and XIIth cranial nerves. It should not be confused with a glomus tumour, which is the only true benign blood vessel tumour (cavernous haemangiomas are dilated blood spaces with thin walls, and port-wine stains/telangiectasias are capillary malformations). Most glomus tumours occur on the upper limbs, especially the digits.

2.38 AD

Klippel–Trenaunay syndrome is characterised by: a cutaneous naevus haemangioma; varicose veins; and bone and soft tissue hypertrophy affecting one or more limbs. There are no pathological arteriovenous fistulas. Venous ulceration should initially be managed by conservative means – as the majority (80%) heal within 1 year – with paste bandages and elastic compression. Stripping of the superficial veins is contraindicated if the deep system is thrombosed. Venous ulceration has a slight gender preponderance – female:male ratio of 2:1. Squamous-cell carcinoma (Marjolin's ulcer) may be seen in long-standing, non-healing venous ulcers.

2.39 CD

Primary lymphoedema is due to a problem of lymphatic development. Secondary lymphoedema is due to causative processes such as trauma, malignant disease, irradiation, infection or inflammation. Anatomically, there are no lymphatic vessels in the epidermis, even in normal subjects. Malignant infiltration of inguinal lymph nodes/lymphatics is a common cause of secondary lymphoedema of the legs. The skin of patients with primary lymphoedema is often hyperkeratotic and thick so that ulceration is uncommon. However, vesicles and fistulas producing pure lymph may occur and are usually successfully treated by conservative measures. Operative treatment is reserved for the rarer resistant cases. In the past, diuretics have been extensively used to treat lymphoedema. However, they are probably of little use because the increased limb volume is composed more of protein and fibrotic tissue than of water.

2.40 Leg ulcers

1. D Postphlebitic

2. C Diabetic

3. A Arterial

Leg ulcers often have multiple aetiologies. The aetiology is usually apparent from taking a clear history and identifying the site of the ulcer. The most common causes of leg ulcers are venous, mixed, arterial, neuropathic, vasculitic (including rheumatoid arthritis) and neoplastic. Venous and postphlebitic ulcers tend to be situated in the gaiter area and have sloping edges.

Arterial ulcers have punched-out edges and often occur at pressure areas at the extremities, e.g. toes. Diabetic ulcers often occur at the site of trauma or ill-fitting shoes. Neoplastic ulcers have raised, rolled or everted edges and may occur anywhere.

2.41 B

Carotid artery stenosis may cause embolisation or thrombotic occlusion leading to transient ischaemic attack, ischaemic stroke or retinal infarct. A patient with asymptomatic carotid stenosis with a reduction in luminal diameter of 50% has a risk of 1–2% per year of developing a stroke. Bruits are an unreliable guide to the presence or severity of carotid stenosis – 37% accuracy for diagnosis of moderate/severe stenosis. Duplex ultrasound may fail to distinguish severe stenosis from occlusion. There is no improved benefit of endarterectomy for stroke prevention in mild/moderate carotid stenosis.

2.42 ABD

Branham's test is where occlusion of the feeding vessel to a large arteriovenous fistula causes bradycardia due to the reversal of the large left to right shunt. AV fistulas deteriorate during puberty and pregnancy. Klippel–Trenaunay syndrome is the combination of cutaneous naevus mesodermal deformities with naevae haemangiomas and lymphatic abnormality: a persistent lateral vein of the thigh giving rise to gross varicose veins but no AV fistula. The Parkes–Weber syndrome consists of multiple AV fistulas leading to limb hypertrophy. AV fistulas can cause embolic events.

2.43 BCDE

5% of patients who undergo endarterectomy for symptomatic carotid stenosis have a stroke or die within 30 days of the operation. Patients are more likely to suffer from perioperative stroke/death if they are female, >75 years, have peripheral vascular disease, a history of cerebral TIA, occlusion of contralateral internal carotid artery or stenosis of the ipsilateral external carotid artery. There is a 3% risk of perioperative myocardial infarction.

2.44 ABDE

Raynaud's syndrome usually affects young women (60–90%) and causes intermittent cold and blue extremities, usually of the fingers. This may lead to trophic finger changes and even gangrene. Raynaud's phenomenon may be primary (Raynaud's disease) or secondary. Secondary causes include connective tissue disorders: systemic lupus erythematosus (SLE), CREST syndrome (calcinosis, Raynaud's phenomenon, [o]esophageal involvement, sclerodactyly, telangiectasia), polyarteritis nodosa (PAN), rheumatoid arthritis (RA), arterial disease, vibration injury as well as blood disorders including cold agglutinins and polycythaemia. The condition may also be associated with the contraceptive pill and beta-blockers.

2.45 CD

These are benign tumours of blood vessels which are most commonly found in the finger or nailbed. Glomus tumours are typically bluish in colour. They are equally common in men and women. They are extremely painful. Subungual tumours can be difficult to detect but may cause rarefaction of the distal phalanx on X-ray. The treatment of glomus tumours is surgical excision.

2.46 BCE

Varicose ulcers are commonly found on the medial side of the lower limb. Venous hypertension secondary to venous stasis leads to extravasation of fibrin from capillaries. The formed fibrin sheath is thought (i.e. fibrin-cuff theory) to block the oxygen diffusion so the skin is relatively ischaemic and ultimately necroses.

Women are more commonly affected than men, usually >40 years of age. Malignant change (Marjolin's ulcer) does occur on the edge of chronic ulcers.

2.47 ACD

Detection of thrombosis by [^{125}I]fibrinogen was first used in 1960. It is incorporated into a developing thrombus. Before the test is performed, iodine uptake by the thyroid is blocked using potassium iodide. False-positive tests occur due to areas of inflammation, bruising, haematoma, arthritis and fresh wounds. False-negative results occur in ageing thrombi and in proximal or pelvic thrombi. This test is unsuitable following hip or lower limb surgery. The [^{125}I]fibrinogen-uptake test is only used as a research tool.

2.48 BCDFG

Chemodectomas are carotid-body tumours which arise from nests of non-chromaffin paraganglionic cells derived from the neural crest. There is a high incidence in the people of Peru (altitude 2000–5000 m), Mexico City and Colorado. In addition, chemodectomas may be bilateral and have an association with phaeochromocytomas. There is a strong familial tendency. Chemodectomas are non-secretory and rarely metastasise.

2.49 ABCE

Classically, ulcers in the gaiter area of the leg are due to venous disease; however, arterial and diabetic ulcers may present in this region. Other causes include vasculitis (including rheumatoid arthritis and scleroderma), rheumatoid arthritis and allergic reactions. Ergot poisoning causes Raynaud's syndrome but not leg ulcers. Rarer causes of leg ulceration include tuberculosis, syphilis, pyoderma gangrenosum, necrobiosis lipoidica and blood dyscrasias.

2.50 ACD

Lymphoedema is an accumulation of tissue fluid as a result of a defect in the lymphatic system principally affecting the legs (80%). However, it may be found in the arm, face and genitalia. Lymphoedema may be divided into primary (familial) and secondary. Secondary lymphoedema in Western countries is usually the result of surgical excision or radiotherapy to lymph nodes. On a worldwide scale, infection is much more common. The worm *Wuchereria bancrofti* causes filiariasis leading to lymphoedema.

2.51 CDE

'Coralline clot' is a fine granular coral-like mass of platelets deposited on the endothelium, and is otherwise known as 'white thrombus'. 'Propagative clot' is red, slippery, non-adherent, and particularly likely to break up and form emboli. It is otherwise known as 'red thrombus'. Aspirin, not anticoagulants, have an effect on platelet aggregation.

2.52 All true

The VIIth, IXth, Xth and XIIth cranial nerves may be damaged during carotid surgery. Postoperative haematomas may cause stridor. Surgical trauma to the carotid sinus nerve may cause postoperative hypertension. This hypertension is usually self-limiting, though some centres use local anaesthesia as a prophylactic measure.

2.53 BD

Critical leg ischaemia is defined by either of the two following criteria:

1. Persistently recurring rest pain requiring regular, adequate analgesia for more than 2 weeks with an ankle systolic pressure of < 50 mmHg, and/or a toe systolic pressure of < 30 mmHg.
2. Ulceration or gangrene of the foot or toes with an ankle systolic pressure of < 50 mmHg and/or a toe systolic pressure of < 30 mmHg.

Critically ischaemic legs due to distal occlusion or embolisation may be treated with thrombolysis (using streptokinase or tissue plasminogen activator). However, since thrombolysis may take several hours to take effect, a clinical decision has to be made regarding whether one can wait this length of time before an irreversible situation is reached. Lumbar sympathectomy may help patients with mild rest pain. It is, however, ineffective once frank gangrene is present.

2.54 Site of arterial disease

1. A Lower aorta

2. H Right superficial femoral artery

The heavy smoker is most likely to have an aortic occlusion causing impaired flow to the internal iliac arteries (Leriche's syndrome).

The diabetic patient is most likely to have a right superficial femoral artery occlusion.

2.55 ABD

Naevus flammeus (salmon patch) is the common birthmark, and appears as a flat pink, red or purple patch, most commonly on the face and neck of newborns. Most involute by 1 year. Port-wine stains are a variant of naevus flammeus, but these lesions grow with the child, becoming elevated and unsightly. They show little or no tendency to regress with time. Spider naevi comprise a small cutaneous arteriole from which small venules radiate. They are common in pregnancy and liver failure. Juvenile haemangiomas usually undergo a rapid growth phase over several months to produce the protruding strawberry naevus. They subsequently regress, and most involute to a small brown spot by the age of 7 years. Cavernous haemangiomas tend to grow with time and rarely involute.

2.56 ABCD

Congenital lymphoedema is caused by abnormality of the superficial lymphatics and is more common in women. It often does not manifest until the third or fourth decade. Lymphovenous anastomosis depends on dilated distal lymphatics, possibly after a radical groin dissection. The Charles' or Homan's operations, which remove the oedematous subcutaneous tissue, have a limited but specific role in the management of lymphoedema.

2.57 ABC

As it leaves the cubital region, the radial artery passes medial to the biceps tendon, and superficial to the insertion of the pronator teres muscle. At the wrist, the artery passes across the floor of the anatomical 'snuff box' over the trapezium, and enters the hand between the two heads of the first dorsal interosseous and the oblique and transverse heads of the adductor pollicis muscles, continuing as the deep palmar arch. The arch is completed medially by a branch of the ulnar artery and allows for anastomosis between these two arteries.

2.58 ABD

An abdominal aneurysm may rupture or cause embolisation. They can be identified by screening programmes and there is current interest in endovascular stenting. Presently, only certain configurations of AAA can be successfully stented. Extension of the aneurysm above the renal arteries precludes stenting. Current practice is to defer operative intervention until the maximum diameter is at least 5.5 cm. The UK small aneurysm trial (1998) reported no survival benefit for early operation in patients with small (4.0–5.5 cm) aortic aneurysms. However, clinical decision-making should be strongly guided by patient preferences and explanation of the risks of surgery.

2.59 AD

The patency rate of internal mammary artery grafts is approximately 90% at 10 years. Vein grafts anastomosed at the same locations have a 10-year patency rate of only about 40%. A major factor predictive of outcome is left ventricular function, and this is thought to be more important than the age of the patient or the number of grafts performed. Predictive risk scores are used in cardiac surgery (e.g. Parsonnet) to give an estimated risk. The score is based on age, ejection fraction, previous CVA, number of diseased vessels, diabetes mellitus, etc. Failure of internal mammary graft function is usually a technical problem and occurs early. Long-term failure of vein grafts is due to intimal proliferation and atheroma deposition.

2.60 C

A glomus tumour is a benign tumour of blood vessels. It lies in the skin, two-thirds are found in the upper limb but they may also arise on the trunk. Half the glomus tumours develop in the digits and one-third subungally. Only 2% of glomus tumours are painless. Treatment is by surgical excision.

2.61 BDE

Nitric oxide (NO), previously known as 'endothelial-derived relaxing factor', is released from endothelial cells. It produces relaxation of vascular smooth muscle and vasodilatation, and is an inhibitor of platelet aggregation. Endotoxin causes a release of NO from the endothelium, and its solubility allows free diffusion.

2.62 BCDE

Diabetic foot ulcers are classically painless as patients often have an associated peripheral neuropathy. The ankle brachial Doppler pressure index is high due to calcification of the vessels. Due to peripheral neuropathy a distorted foot (Charcot joints) are seen and amputations (autoamputation and/or surgical amputation) are common.

2.63 All true

An arteriovenous fistula (AVF) represents a low-resistance pathway for blood flow. The resistance is less in a side-to-side AVF than in an 'H-shaped' AVF. Blood flow in the proximal artery is always increased but may be imperceptible when the fistula is small. On the other hand, blood pressure in the distal artery usually decreases. Central compensatory mechanisms are brought into play, including an increase in heart rate, stroke volume, cardiac output and blood volume. Several anatomical changes have been noted in both the arterial and venous sides of the AVF. The artery tends to elongate and distend with time and may even become aneurysmal.

2.64 ABDE

The femoral (Scarpa's) triangle is a fascial space in the upper medial thigh. Its sides are formed superiorly by the inguinal ligament, medially by adductor longus and laterally by sartorius. The floor is formed by the iliopsoas, pectineus and adductor longus. The triangle contains the femoral vessels and nerve. Within the femoral triangle, the femoral artery divides into its deep and superficial branches, while the femoral vein receives deep femoral and saphenous tributaries.

2.65 D

Leg ulcers result in the loss of 500,000 working days/year in the UK and an annual expenditure on treatment of about £50 million. Pure venous ulcers are the most common type, but the routine use of Doppler ultrasound has shown that about 10% of these are accompanied by previously unrecognised arterial disease. Venous ulcers tend to have a shallow base with a flat margin and often coexist with signs of chronic venous hypertension such as lipodermatosclerosis and atrophie blanche. Ischaemic ulcers are commonly painful, deep and accompanied by dependent rubor, skin pallor and poor venous filling. Skin cancers make up 2% of leg ulcers and the suspicion of malignancy should be raised by the presence of rolled irregular edges and exuberant granulation tissue. Ulcers may be colonised by a range of bacteria which can be successfully eradicated by cleansing and the removal of slough. Topical antibiotics are best avoided, but systemic antibiotics are indicated in the treatment of periulcer cellulitis.

2.66 A

Abdominal aortic aneurysms (AAA) occur about 4 times more commonly in males. The incidence of aortic aneurysms is rising in Western countries. They can be safely treated by observation if asymptomatic and <5.5 cm in size. Above this size, the risk of rupture rises exponentially and patients are offered surgery if they are fit enough to tolerate the procedure. The operative mortality for ruptured aneurysms remains at least 50%, and for elective surgery <5%. 98% of AAA are infrarenal. Only 5% of AAA are suitable for abdominal tube stenting. Bifurcated grafts allow up to 40% of AAA to be stented.

The popliteal artery is the commonest site for true aneurysm formation apart from the aorta. 10% of patients with AAA have a popliteal artery aneurysm, and 40% of patients with popliteal artery aneurysms have an AAA.

2.67 Carotid artery disease

1. D Right carotid endarterectomy

2. B MRI head

3. D Right carotid endarterectomy

Patients with carotid territory TIAs, amaurosis fugax or a stroke (with subsequent recovery), and a >70% stenosis should be offered endarterectomy. The risks of the operation are less than the risk of suffering a disabling stroke, providing the operation is performed within 6 months of the stroke. Endarterectomy should carry a mortality of <2%, and a 1–2%

risk of stroke. It is normally too late to operate on completely occluded veins. Patients with lesser degrees of stenosis should be given antiplatelet drug therapy.

A young patient with optic neuritis and foot drop should first have an MRI scan of the brain to look for demyelinating disease.

2.68 Varicose veins

1. A Varicose vein surgery

2. C Elevation and NSAIDs

3. B IV heparin

Varicose veins must be dealt with surgically if they are responsible for causing an ulcerating lesion that is bleeding intermittently – this should be done promptly.

Episodes of thrombophlebitis are best treated by elevation, analgesics (NSAIDs are useful) and external elastic support.

On confirmation of a DVT, patients should be started on intravenous heparin as soon as possible. Intravenous heparin has been the mainstay of treatment; now, however, patients are frequently treated with low-molecular-weight heparins on an outpatient basis, before starting warfarin therapy. Warfarin therapy aims to prevent the formation of clots; heparin aims to prevent their propagation and dispersal.

2.69 Lower limb ischaemia

1. A Surgical embolectomy

2. C Angioplasty

3. B Femoropopliteal bypass graft

The first patient is likely to have had a mural thrombus post MI that has embolised to his leg. He may also have been in atrial fibrillation previously. As he has critical ischaemia, surgical embolectomy is indicated.

Angioplasty is useful for short stenoses. This has better results for proximal stenosis above the inguinal ligament. Angioplasty for occluded vessels is now possible in specialist centres using cutting-balloon or subintimal angioplasty techniques.

A patient with rest pain has critical ischaemia and needs urgent intervention. A 10 cm stenosis is too long for a successful angioplasty. A good distal run-off would allow distal bypass grafting. The SFA is the commonest site for lower limb atherosclerosis because the vessel narrows as it passes through the adductor hiatus.

ANSWERS – CHAPTER 3: HEAD, NECK, ENDOCRINE AND PAEDIATRIC

3.1 ACDE

The submandibular gland is a lobulated gland made up of a superficial and a deep part, which are continuous with each other around the posterior border of the mylohyoid muscle. The gland is partly infralateral, enclosed in an investing layer of deep cervical fascia, platysma muscle and skin. Laterally it is crossed by the cervical branch of the facial nerve and vein. The facial artery is related to the posterior and superior aspects of the superficial part of the gland.

3.2 Anatomy of joints in the head and neck

1. B Temporomandibular

2. G Atlantoaxial

3. F Cricoarytenoid

The temporomandibular joint has a fibrocartilagenous disc within it.

The atlantoaxial joint is stabilised by a transverse ligament which holds the odontoid process in register with a facet on the anterior arch of the atlas.

The cricoarytenoid joints are typical saddle joints allowing rotatory and gliding movements over the shoulders of the posterior arch of the cricoid cartilage.

3.3 B

Three types of papillae are present on the upper surface of the anterior two-thirds of the tongue, namely: filiform, fungiform and (circum)vallate papillae. The mucous membrane covering the posterior one-third of the tongue is devoid of papillae but has a nodular irregular surface caused by the presence of underlying lymphatic tissue, the lingual tonsil.

3.4 AE

The clavipectoral fascia arises from the clavicle and encloses the pectoralis minor before fusing with the floor of the axilla. The thoracodorsal nerve supplies the latissimus dorsi. Damage to the long thoracic nerve (serratus anterior) causes a winged scapula. Level I nodes lie lateral to pectoralis minor, level II behind and level III medial to the pectoralis minor. Division of the intercostobrachial nerve (T2) can lead to anaesthesia on the medial upper arm.

3.5 BDE

The superior thyroid artery arises from the external carotid artery and enters the upper pole of the thyroid gland close to the external laryngeal nerve, which supplies the cricothyroid muscle, a tensor of the vocal cord. Damage to this nerve causes the loss of high-pitched phonation. The inferior thyroid artery, absent in 5%, arises from the thyrocervical trunk of the subclavian artery. The former should be ligated as far laterally as possible to avoid damaging the recurrent laryngeal nerve. Damage to one recurrent laryngeal nerve causes a weakened voice, damage to both causes semiadduction and respiratory difficulties. The isthmus is normally in front of the second and third tracheal rings, although variations are common.

3.6 ACE

The thyroid gland lies deep to the myofascial layer (strap muscles and investing layer of deep cervical fascia), closely applied to the thyroid and cricoid cartilages. The gland initially moves up on swallowing before returning to its normal position. The thyroid gland is highly vascular, normally accounting for 5% of cardiac output. While the superior thyroid artery is a branch of the external carotid artery, the inferior thyroid artery arises from the subclavian artery, via the thyrocervical trunk. There may also be a 'thyroidea IMA' artery that may arise from the aortic arch, brachiocephalic or even internal mammary. The thyroid venous plexus usually drains via 3 pairs of veins: the superior and middle thyroid veins drain into the internal jugular, the inferior thyroid veins drain into the brachiocephalic vein.

3.7 DE

The Eustachian (auditory) tube connects the middle ear with the nasopharynx, opening above the pharyngeal tonsil (adenoid). The eustachian tube equalises air pressure on either side of the tympanic membrane allowing it to move freely. It is shorter and more horizontal in the child. With growth, the tube becomes elongated and gains downward angulation. In the adult, the Eustachian tube is approximately 3.5 cm long. The posterior third is bony, the rest cartilaginous. The bony part of the tube perforates the petrous temporal bone.

3.8 BCEF

The sensory innervation to the tongue is from cranial nerves VII, VIII and IX. The tongue deviates to the side of a CN XII lesion on protrusion, is active during the first stage of swallowing and contains the lingual tonsil in the dorsum of its posterior third. The tongue is retracted up and back by the styloglossus muscle, protruded by genioglossus and depressed by the hyoglossus.

3.9 ABDF

The fibrous capsule of the parotid gland is an upward extension of the deep investing layer of cervical fascia that attaches to the zygomatic arch. The medial wall of the capsule is separated from the carotid sheath by the styloid process and associated muscles (stylopharyngeus, stylohyoid, styloglossus). The external carotid artery passes through the gland, supplying it as it does so. No facial vessels are related to the gland. The facial nerve enters the gland and divides within it into its five terminal branches.

3.10 CDE

The submandibular gland consists of a deep and superficial part. The superficial part lies in the digastric triangle (above and between the two bellies of the digastric muscle). The hypoglossal nerve runs medial to superficial part of the gland. The gland is superficial to the mylohyoid and hyoglossus muscles. One-third of the submandibular gland lies below the lower border of the mandible and two-thirds above it.

3.11 DE

The true vocal folds have a stratified squamous epithelium, innervated by the recurrent laryngeal branch (CN X), and are formed by the vocal ligament (the free edge of the quadrangular membrane forms the false vocal cord). Above the vocal cords, the larynx is sensorily innervated by the internal laryngeal nerve (CN X). The cords are adducted by the lateral cricoarytenoid muscle, abducted by the posterior cricoarytenoid and tensed by tilting the thyroid cartilage downwards and forwards by contracting the cricothyroid muscle. All the laryngeal muscles are supplied by the recurrent laryngeal nerve except for cricothyroid, which is supplied by the external laryngeal nerve.

3.12 BC

The great auricular nerve turns upwards round the lateral border of the sternocleidomastoid muscle outside the triangle. The posterior belly of the omohyoid muscle and its intermediate tendon pass diagonally through the triangle (they are palpable, often confused with both the upper trunk of the brachial plexus and the suprascapular nerve), and the clavicular (intermediate) and acromial (lateral) branches of the supraclavicular nerves course through the roof. Lying medially, outside the triangle, are the roots of the brachial plexus sandwiched between the scalenus posterior and medius muscles. The vertebral artery lies within the pyramidal space inferiorly, before ascending through the foramen transversarium of the C1–C6 vertebrae. Other components of the posterior triangle include the semispinalis capitis, splenius capitis, levator scapulae and scalenus medius muscles and the spinal accessory nerve.

3.13 AF

The axons conveying taste over the anterior two-thirds of the tongue and secretomotor fibres to the submandibular and sublingual salivary glands (the parotid is innervated by CN IX) are found in the chorda tympani nerve. The chorda tympani courses across the tympanic membrane beneath the mucous membrane of the middle ear after leaving the facial canal approximately 0.5 cm above the stylomastoid foramen. It exits the middle ear by passing through the petrotympanic fissure medially, and runs forwards on the medial side of the spine of the sphenoid bone. After entering the infratemporal fossa it merges with the lingual nerve. The chorda tympani, therefore, is not related to the parotid gland. It also escapes injury when the facial nerve is compressed within the most distal part of the facial canal. (The 'facial canal' is the passageway of the facial nerve after it emerges from the internal auditory meatus.)

3.14 ABCD

The pituitary fossa, or sella turcica, lies above the body of the sphenoid bone and its associated sinus. The pituitary fossa can be easily identified on a lateral skull X-ray. The optic chiasma lies above and towards the back of the sella turcica. A pituitary tumour would first impinge on the anterior part of the optic chiasma and so cause a temporal hemianopia.

3.15 C

The recurrent laryngeal nerves are sensory to the subglottic region and supply all the intrinsic muscles except the cricothyroid.

3.16 B

The nasolacrimal duct drains into the inferior meatus; the sphenoidal air sinus into the sphenoethmoidal recess; and the posterior ethmoidal air sinus into the superior meatus. The middle meatus contains the bulla ethmoidalis of the middle ethmoidal air sinus which drains through a hiatus in the bulla. Olfactory epithelium containing the primary olfactory neurones lines the superior nasal recess (roof of the nasal cavity) under cover of the cribriform plate of the ethmoid bone.

3.17 B

The posterior cerebral artery supplies the cerebral peduncle and the optic tract, as well as the inferomedial surface of the temporal and occipital lobes. Occlusion causes a contralateral hemianopia and hemianaesthesia. The posterior cerebral artery supplies the inferolateral surface of the temporal lobe, lateral and medial surfaces of the occipital lobe, the cerebral peduncle and the optic tract. Occlusion of this vessel results in a contralateral homonymous hemianopia.

3.18 BD

60% of branchial cysts occur in men. Although the highest incidence is found in the third decade, they may occur between 1 and 70 years of age. Two-thirds are found on the left, and 2% are bilateral. Two-thirds of the branchial cysts are anterior to the sternocleidomastoid in the upper third of the neck. The most common presenting features are continuous intermittent swelling or pain. Infection only occurs in 15% of cases. The cysts are lined by stratified squamous epithelium. Branchial cysts contain straw-coloured fluid in which cholesterol crystals can be found.

3.19 ABE

80% of salivary gland adenomas arise in the parotid gland. 80% are pleomorphic adenomas and 80% arise in the superficial lobe. Most adenomas present in middle age or later in life, and have an equal sex incidence. Parotid adenomas usually occur in the superficial part of the gland external to the plane of the lower branches of the facial nerve. Occasionally they occur in the deep part of the gland. A parotid adenoma is a benign tumour and does not impinge on the nerves to cause a facial palsy. Frey's syndrome is a late complication of parotidectomy, occurring in as many as 25% of patients. It results from the division of the parasympathetic secretory motor fibres originally innervating the gland. These nerve fibres regenerate in the skin where they assume control of sweat gland activity. Facial sweating then occurs in response to salivatory stimuli (gustatory sweating).

3.20 Laryngeal cancer

1. **A Total laryngectomy and neck dissection**
2. **B Radiotherapy**
3. **F Excision of vocal cord mucosa**
4. **D Hemilaryngectomy (vertical)**
5. **E Supraglottic laryngectomy (horizontal) and neck dissection**

The tumour stage in the first scenario is T_3N_{2a}. Partial laryngectomy is inadequate, therefore total laryngectomy combined with neck dissection is the surgical treatment of choice. Radiotherapy may be given postoperatively. Chemotherapy is indicated for inoperable disease.

Radiotherapy is as effective as surgery in the treatment of T_1 tumours. However, the resulting voice quality is better than after surgery.

Close monitoring is required following removal of a carcinoma in situ.

Vertical laryngectomy is more appropriate in the fourth case due to the increased risk of cartilage involvement.

Nodal metastases are found in 55% of supraglottic tumours. Therefore radical neck dissection or both is often required for large supraglottic tumours.

3.21 Lumps in the neck

1. **A Cystic hygroma**
2. **D Branchial cyst**
3. **E Cervical lymphadenopathy**

A cystic hygroma is a congenital cystic lymphatic malformation at the root of the neck, 50% of which are present at birth. They are thin-walled and transilluminate. CT and MRI may be helpful in determining their extent.

Branchial cysts usually present in the third decade. Patients complain of an enlarging lump usually presenting from behind the junction of the upper and middle thirds of the anterior border of the sternocleidomastoid, though it may occur behind the muscle. Sternomastoid tumours occur in neonates and tend to disappear as the patient grows and the abnormal muscle becomes fibrotic – leading to torticollis.

Posterior triangle lumps are usually lymph nodes. Other causes include pharyngeal pouches, cystic hygromas and subclavian aneurysms.

3.22 ACDE

Maxillary sinus carcinoma tend to affect African, Japanese and Arabic populations. It is much rarer in Western Europe and America. 90% of cancers of the sinuses affect the maxillary and ethmoidal sinuses, with only 10% affecting the frontal and sphenoidal sinuses. Definite risk factors include dust from hardwood and nickel. Other factors implicated are radiation, mustard gas production and materials used in boot making. Clinical features include nasal obstruction, epistaxis, toothache, loosening of teeth, destruction of bone (which may lead to proptosis and diplopia), invasion of nerves causing numbness of the facial palate and invasion of the infratemporal fossa causing trismus. 10% of cases have metastatic lymph node involvement at presentation.

3.23 CG

The frontal nerve arises from the ophthalmic division of the trigeminal nerve in the lateral wall of the cavernous sinus. It enters the orbits through the superior orbital fissure. Just before it reaches the orbital margin it divides into the supratrochlear and supraorbital nerves. The supraorbital nerve passes through the supraorbital foramen, and supplies the skin of the forehead. The ophthalmic artery branches off the internal carotid artery at the cavernous sinus, and passes through the optic canal with the optic nerve. The optic nerve is surrounded by a sheath of pia, arachnoid and dura mater. The nasociliary nerve arises from the ophthalmic division of the trigeminal nerve in the lateral fourth of the cavernous sinus, and enters the orbit through the superior orbital fissure within the tendinous ring. The branches of the nasociliary nerve supply the ethmoidal sinuses, sphenoidal sinuses, skin of the upper eyelids and nose. The inferior ramus of the oculomotor nerve gives off branches to the inferior rectus, medial rectus and the inferior oblique muscles. The superior ramus of the oculomotor nerves supplies the levator palpebrae superioris, thus may give rise to a ptosis if cut.

3.24 A

There are very few distinct characteristics of a malignant thyroid nodule and hence ultrasound, fine-needle aspiration and cytology are required. Benign enlargement of the thyroid itself may compress or displace any of its close relations such as the trachea and oesophagus, thus leading to stridor and dysphagia. A carcinoma of the thyroid would invade its neighbouring structures rather than displace them, eroding into the trachea, oesophagus and adjacent carotid sheath. In cases of a malignant thyroid nodule, the recurrent laryngeal nerve and cervical sympathetic chain may be involved so producing hoarseness and Horner's syndrome respectively.

3.25 AD

Saliva is always hypotonic to plasma. The pH of saliva from resting glands is slightly acidic. During active secretion, however, the saliva becomes more basic, and its pH increases to nearly 8.

The concentration of potassium in saliva is always much greater than its concentration in plasma. When salivary flow rates are very low, salivary potassium levels are high.

The serous acinar cells have zymogen granules that contain salivary amylase – major digestive function of saliva – which breaks down starch.

3.26 Congenital neck lumps

1. A Laryngocele

2. B Thyroglossal cyst

Laryngoceles are laryngeal saccules that are expanded with air. They may occur after prolonged straining – e.g. by wind instrument players. They may be internal (presenting in the false cords) or external, presenting as a neck lump.

A thyroglossal cyst is a remnant of the thyroglossal duct which has not obliterated. Surgical treatment is by Sistrunk's operation (involving removal of the cyst as well as the thyroglossal tract from the back of the tongue to and including the middle third of the hyoid bone).

3.27 AC

Glue ear is a serous viscus effusion that may occur after an episode of acute otitis media. Conditions predisposing to the condition are Eustachian tube dysfunction, adenoidal hypertrophy and allergic conditions. Cleft palate has no association.

3.28 CD

The vast majority of piriform fossa tumours are squamous in origin, and may be visualised by indirect laryngoscopy and fibre-optic endoscopy. These tumours usually grow silently, and commonly present with cervical lymphadenopathy. However, they may occasionally cause referred pain to the ear. Radiotherapy is of little value in their treatment and surgery is the only real hope of cure.

3.29 B

Earache from acute tonsillitis is due to referred pain along the glossopharyngeal nerve which runs in the tonsillar bed, and which sends a tympanic branch to the tympanic plexus in the middle ear. The other nerves are not involved.

3.30 AC

Timolol is a beta-blocker, used in the first-line treatment of chronic simple glaucoma. It probably acts by reducing the rate of aqueous humour production.

Pilocarpine and adrenaline are second-line treatments for the same condition. Pilocarpine acts by opening up inefficient drainage channels in the trabecular meshwork, which have been caused by contraction of the ciliary muscle. Adrenaline acts by increasing outflow through the trabecular meshwork and by reducing the rate of production of aqueous humour.

Local anaesthetics, such as tetracaine (amethocaine), have no effect on the pupil, whilst opioids cause pupillary constriction.

3.31 B

A right homonymous hemianopia would result from a left occipital lobe infarction and the macular would also be affected. Right eye blindness is seen when the right optic nerve is injured. The lateral rectus muscle is supplied by the VIth (abducent) cranial nerve whose nucleus is in the caudal part of the pons.

3.32 BC

Bilateral vocal cord paralysis is a recognised complication of thyroidectomy, and is caused by damage to the recurrent laryngeal nerves. In a partial unilateral paralysis of the recurrent laryngeal nerve, the cords lie in the midline. A complete recurrent laryngeal paralysis would cause the cords to lie midway between the normal resting position and the midline. Patients must therefore be assessed immediately for airway obstruction which manifests as stridor. In this instance, prompt re-intubation is indicated. In the longer term, laser arytenoidectomy provides the best compromise between a patent airway and functional voice. Diphtheria may cause upper airway obstruction, but does so by the production of a thick fibrinopurulent film over the lumen.

3.33 ACDE

Tracheostomy can produce perichondritis and subglottic stenosis if the cricoid cartilage is injured; therefore the surgical approach should be below the first cartilage ring, preferably through rings 3 and 4. Partial dislodgement may lead to erosion of the innominate artery, producing catastrophic haemorrhage. Tube changing should be avoided till 3 days after surgery, until a track is well established and the tube can be easily changed.

3.34 All true

Other complications include pneumothorax, dislodgement of the tube (partial or complete), obstruction of the tube or trachea, tracheal stenosis, sepsis, haemorrhage, cuff prolapse and intubation granuloma of the vocal cords. Subglottic stenosis occurs if the tracheal rings 1 and 2 are damaged.

3.35 ACE

The structures to be avoided at the time of submandibular gland excision include: the mandibular branch of the facial nerve; the hypoglossal and lingual nerves; and the facial artery and retromandibular vein. Linguinal nerve damage results in ipsilateral anaesthesia and hemiplegia of the tongue. Hypoglossal nerve injury restricts the mobility of the tongue. Frey's syndrome (gustatory sweating) is a complication of parotid surgery.

3.36 ABD

80% of parotid tumours are benign and 80% of these are pleomorphic adenomas. 15% of salivary gland neoplasms are found in the submandibular gland. A proportion of tumours are slow growing, but should not be biopsied as they are at risk of tumour-seeding along the tract. Otalgia (referred pain) may be a presenting feature.

3.37 Thyroid disease

1. B Recurrent thyroid lymphoma
2. D Early anaplastic carcinoma
3. A Hot nodule in the thyroid gland
4. C Follicular adenoma
5. E Follicular carcinoma

A solitary, hot, functioning nodule is known as Plummer's syndrome and accounts for only 5% of all cases of thyrotoxicosis.

Follicular adenomas only require resection.

However, if the histology demonstrates a carcinoma, a completion thyroidectomy with radio-iodine treatment is carried out. It is impossible to differentiate follicular adenoma and carcinoma if follicular cells are seen following fine-needle aspiration of the thyroid gland. A partial thyroidectomy is therefore necessary to examine histologically if the capsule has been invaded (carcinoma).

Lymphoma of the thyroid is treated by surgery followed by radiotherapy to the neck and mediastinum. Chemotherapy is added to treatment if distant metastases or recurrent disease is present.

3.38 ABC

Ludwig's angina is a severe spreading cellulitis (infection of the submandibular, sublingual and submental spaces) caused by a beta-haemolytic streptococcus. It is usually caused by dental sepsis. It may cause dyspnoea, dysphagia and dysphonia. The priority is to secure the airway and treat with intravenous antibiotics. The infected spaces should be decompressed and the infected tooth removed.

3.39 E

The two main aetiological factors for cancer of the oral cavity are excessive smoking and alcohol consumption. Men are more commonly affected and the median age of presentation is 60 years. The most common signs and symptoms are an ulcer, swelling, pain and a neck lump. The tumours usually arise in the salivary gutters of the mouth. Indications for surgery are failed radiotherapy, bony invasion and cervical metastasis. Chemotherapy has little role in the management of oral cavity malignancy.

3.40 DE

The anterior division of Vc has one sensory branch (the buccal nerve to the skin of the cheek and mucosa of the vestibule). All other branches are motor to the muscles of mastication, i.e. the masseter, temporalis and lateral pterygoid. The lower jaw teeth are supplied by the inferior alveolar branch of the posterior division of Vc. The buccinator muscle is supplied by VII. Unopposed contraction of the contralateral lateral pterygoid muscle deviates the jaw to the side of the lesion during protrusion. None of the muscles of the pharynx are supplied by the anterior division of Vc, so dysphagia is not a feature of damage to this nerve.

3.41 CD

Epistaxis results from a wide range of local and systemic conditions. It may be a presenting feature of haematological disease, e.g. leukaemia or lymphoma. The most common site of epistaxis is the anterior nasal septum (Little's area). If bleeding does not stop with pressure, then packing (anteronasal or postnasal) is required. A Foley urinary catheter, not a Fogarty catheter, is useful for staunching the haemorrhage. Sedation should be avoided as this may compromise respiration.

3.42 AD

Lateral swellings of the neck include lymph nodes, salivary glands, branchial cysts, cervical ribs, carotid body tumours (chemodectomas), cystic hygromas, sternocleidomastoid tumours, arteriovenous fistulas and lateral thyroid lobe lesions.

3.43 A

Acute otitis media is very common especially in children, in whom presentation may be in the form of generalised malaise, pyrexia or GI upset. Otalgia and hearing loss are more common features in adults. The causative organisms are usually *Streptococcus pneumoniae* or *S. haemophilus.* The first-line treatment is a broad-spectrum antibiotic, e.g. amoxicillin. Myringotomy is only advocated once perforation has occurred. If the acute phase does not settle, a more chronic infection develops and in rare instances a cholesteatoma may form.

3.44 CD

The head is turned using the contralateral sternocleidomastoid muscle, stimulated by impulses passing in the spinal accessory nerve. The movement takes place at the atlantoaxial joint about a vertical axis through the odontoid process of the axis, and is limited by the vertical alignment of the two attachments of the contralateral sternocleidomastoid muscle (contralateral mastoid process and sternoclavicular joint).

3.45 ABC

The optic nerve and retina are part of the CNS. The optic nerve is invested by all meningeal layers. Since the central retinal artery travels in the optic nerve after branching off the ophthalmic artery, damage to the optic nerve commonly causes retinal infarction. Ptosis is a feature of both IIIrd nerve lesions and Horner's syndrome. The afferent arc of the corneal reflex is the nasociliary branch of Va. Blow-out fractures of the orbit either detach the suspensory ligament of the eye, or entrap the recti muscles, usually the inferior rectus muscle; both conditions are associated with diplopia.

3.46 CD

Salivary gland calculi are most commonly found in the submandibular gland (80% cases) and are associated with a high pH and higher mucus content. They most commonly occur in the fourth and fifth decades. Calculi are associated with chronic sialadenitis, diabetes mellitus, hypertension and chronic liver disease. Only 20% of submandibular and 60% of parotid stones are visible on X-ray.

3.47 All true

Middle ear infection is one of the commonest sources of a brain abscess (temporal, cerebellum). This may subsequently give rise to clinical features of raised intracranial pressure, cranial neuropathies (III–VII) and visual disturbance. Sudden deafness may be caused by middle ear effusion.

3.48 BDE

Fracture of the maxilla may occur at three levels: Le Fort I, II and III. A Le Fort III fracture is the most severe and is the result of separation of the mid-facial skeleton from the anterior cranial base. Dental malocclusion is associated with displaced fractures. Le Fort II and III fractures cause features of orbital and nasoethmoidal fractures. The characteristic clinical features of a Le Fort III fracture are: panda eyes, gross mid-facial swelling, CSF rhinorrhoea, bilateral epistaxis and dental malocclusion. Only undisplaced fractures are treated conservatively.

3.49 BC

Swellings of the neck considered to be midline include thyroglossal cysts, pharyngeal pouches, plunging ranulas, subhyoid bursas, laryngoceles and lesions in the thyroid isthmus.

3.50 BCDE

The headache associated with intracranial tumours is most noticeable in the early morning, often exacerbated by movement or coughing. Change in behaviour, mood or degree of alertness may be reported by the patient's relatives or friends. Partial IIIrd and IVth cranial nerve palsies occur with incipient brain herniation at the tentorial notch – patients complain of diplopia on lateral gaze. An apnoeic attack is a rare presenting feature of an intracranial tumour, but occurs where there is a sudden brain herniation with coning at the tentorium or foramen magnum. Early morning headache and vomiting is a well recognised feature.

3.51 ADF

The most common presentation of papillary carcinoma is a thyroid nodule. 85% of irradiation-induced tumours are papillary. Children and young adults (10–20 years of age) are the population at greatest risk. It is medullary carcinoma which secretes calcitonin. Papillary carcinoma spreads to the paratracheal and cervical lymph nodes. It is frequently multifocal (30–87%) and rarely encapsulated. Blood-borne spread is usually a late feature. It is a slow-growing tumour with a good prognosis.

3.52 BCE

Unilateral vocal fold paralysis does not cause respiratory distress on its own. Patients may not notice the vocal effects unless they have a trained voice. Tracheomalacia (softening of the trachea) may lead to tracheal collapse. The treatment for this is intubation.

3.53 E

Men (aged 60–70 years) are affected significantly more frequently than women, with a ratio of 6:1. Most laryngeal carcinomas develop on the vocal folds. Progressive voice change is the earliest sign. Stridor and dyspnoea are late features. Examination is performed by indirect laryngoscopy. Microlaryngoscopy is helpful when views are difficult or when a biopsy is needed. Radiotherapy alone may suppress local symptoms. In advanced disease, radical radiotherapy is required. Curative treatment usually involves radiotherapy, surgery, or a combination of the two.

3.54 ACD

The transverse cervical nerve emerges as a single trunk behind the posterior border of the sternocleidomastoid and is superficial to the muscle. The transverse cervical artery is found in the posterior triangle of the neck just above the clavicle. The great auricular nerve (C2–C3), is a large trunk that passes vertically upwards over the sternocleidomastoid. The external jugular vein commences behind the angle of the mandible, formed by the union of the posterior auricular vein and the posterior division of the retromandibular vein. It descends obliquely across to the sternocleidomastoid and drains into the subclavian vein.

3.55 ABE

The inferior thyroid artery is a branch of the thyrocervical trunk which arises from the subclavian artery. The inferior thyroid artery supplies the inferior pole of the thyroid gland and gives off oesophageal branches. In addition, it supplies both the superior and inferior parathyroid glands. The course of the inferior thyroid artery is closely related to the recurrent laryngeal nerve; and hence in a thyroidectomy, it is preferable to ligate the artery lateral to the gland to avoid neural damage.

3.56 ABCE

The structures passing through the foramen magnum include the: medulla oblongata; meninges; spinal parts of the accessory nerves; meningeal branches of the upper cervical nerves; vertebral arteries; and anterior and posterior spinal arteries.

3.57 All true

The three compartments of the jugular foramen are: the anterior, containing the inferior petrosal sinus and CN IX; the middle, containing CN X and CN XI; and the posterior, containing the internal jugular vein as a continuation of the sigmoid sinus. The inferior petrosal sinus drains the cavernous sinus, leaving the skull via the jugular foramen and draining into the superior bulb of the internal jugular vein. The internal jugular descends the neck in the anterior of the carotid sheath, and drains into the brachiocephalic vein on each side behind the sternoclavicular joint. The ansa loops anteriorly around the carotid sheath under cover of the sternocleidomastoid.

3.58 All false

The superior vena cava (SVC) drains all structures above the diaphragm except the heart and lungs. It also receives the azygos vein which drains the lumbar and subcostal regions. The SVC is formed behind the first costal cartilage by the union of the right and left brachiocephalic veins. It ends behind the third costal cartilage as it enters the right atrium. The SVC has no valves. The thoracic duct drains into the left brachiocephalic vein (or sometimes into the subclavian or internal jugular vein).

3.59 BCEF

The ophthalmic artery is a branch of the internal carotid and enters the orbit through the optic foramen. The ophthalmic artery then crosses the optic nerve to the medial side of the orbit accompanied by the nasociliary nerve. The supraorbital and nasal arteries are two branches of the ophthalmic artery that supply part of the skin of the forehead. The central retinal artery is the first and smallest branch of the ophthalmic artery. The cornea is avascular.

3.60 BD

The carotid artery divides into the external and internal carotid branches at the upper border of the thyroid cartilage. The external carotid artery is deep to the hypoglossal nerve having been crossed by it at the level of the hyoid bone. The carotid sinus is normally found at the division of the common carotid artery or at the commencement of the internal carotid artery.

3.61 AB

The spinal canal is anterior to the ligamentum flavum but posterior to the vertebral disc. The spinal cord ends at L1.

3.62 AC

The thoracic duct leaves the cysterna chyli at the level of L1–L2, ascends into the thorax to the right of the descending thoracic aorta, crosses the midline gradually to reach the left border of the oesophagus (plane of Louis, T4), where it continues to run upwards reaching the root of the neck. It then curves behind the carotid sheath and arches over the left subclavian artery to drain into the left brachiocephalic vein, although it can also drain into the other adjacent major veins. It carries lymph from the lower limbs, abdominal and pelvic regions, left thorax, left head and neck plus the left arm.

3.63 All false

A pharyngeal pouch (Zenker's diverticulum) represents a pulsion diverticulum that protrudes from the back of the pharynx into Killian's dehiscence just above the cricopharyngeus. It is more common in elderly people or patients of middle age. Patients (3:1 male to female) usually complain of regurgitation, gurgling noises and recurrent chest infections. Progressive dysphagia, halitosis and aspiration pneumonia may also occur. The diagnosis is best confirmed by barium swallow. Endoscopy is unnecessary and carries a risk of iatrogenic perforation. Treatment is by excision of the diverticulum and closure of the defect in two layers. This is preferably combined with cricopharyngeal myomectomy. Left-sided pouches are more common than right-sided ones.

3.64 BCDE

Pharyngeal webs are more common in women and may be part of the Plummer–Vinson (Patterson–Kelly) syndrome where the patient also has an associated iron deficiency anaemia giving rise to a microcytic picture. This is a premalignant condition. Webs will also increase the incidence and risk of aspiration.

3.65 Calcium metabolism

1. **C Tertiary hyperparathyroidism**
2. **A Primary hyperparathyroidism**
3. **B Secondary hyperparathyroidism**
4. **E Hypoparathyroidism**

Hyperparathyroidism is primarily caused by an adenoma (80% of cases). The remaining causes are due to hyperplasia (19%) or carcinoma (1%).

Secondary hyperparathyroidism is due to a chronic calcium deficiency, usually as a result of chronic renal impairment.

Tertiary disease occurs when the parathyroid glands become autonomous as a result of long-standing and sustained positive feedback by low free-ionised calcium concentrations.

3.66 Treatment of thyrotoxicosis
1. B Carbimazole
2. A Propranolol
3. D Subtotal thyroidectomy

Thyrotoxicosis is managed conservatively in the first instance.
Propanolol, a beta-blocker, is good for reducing anxiety and for the treatment of cardiac arrhythmias such as atrial fibrillation.
Care must be taken when prescribing carbimazole as blood dyscrasias occur in 2% of cases. The treatment for thyrotoxicosis which has not responded to medical treatment is subtotal thyroidectomy.

3.67 Familial endocrine disease
1. A MEN-1 syndrome
2. A MEN-1 syndrome
3. E Hyperparathyroidism

The multiple endocrine neoplasia (MEN) syndromes are inherited in an autosomal dominant manner or occur as new mutations. MEN-1 consists of pituitary adrenal cortex, pancreatic islet cell (gastrinomas, insulinomas) and parathyroid adenomas or hyperplasia. Patients with MEN-2A and -2B develop phaeochromocytomas and medullary thyroid carcinomas. In addition, those with MEN-2A develop parathyroid hyperplasia but are phenotypically normal, while those with MEN-2B tend to be marfanoid and develop submucosal neuromas.

3.68 ADE

There are numerous causes of raised serum calcium levels. The most common include metastatic bony tumour deposits, primary hyperparathyroidism and multiple myeloma. Secondary hyperparathyroidism occurs in response to a low serum calcium level. Tertiary hyperparathyroidism is most commonly seen in chronic renal failure. Other causes of hypercalcaemia include thyrotoxicosis, Paget's disease of bone, sarcoidosis, vitamin D intoxication, Addison's disease, thiazide diuretics, TB and familial hypocalciuric hypercalcaemia.

3.69 Paediatric investigations

1. A A 'double-bubble sign' on plain AXR
2. D Intramural gas on plain AXR
3. F A 'target' lesion on abdominal ultrasound
4. B A 'cone' on contrast enema

Persistent bile-stained vomiting (if the atresia is distal to the second part where the common bile duct enters the duodenum) in a newborn infant may indicate a diagnosis of duodenal atresia. The typical radiological feature is the 'double-bubble' seen on plain AXR (an air-filled dilated stomach and first part of duodenum, creating two discrete air shadows).

A premature baby presenting with bile-stained vomiting and rectal bleeding is at high risk of suffering from necrotising enterocolitis. The typical radiological feature of this condition is gas within the bowel wall on plain AXR. It may be associated with gas in the portal system and/or free air in the abdomen when the disease progresses to intestinal perforation.

An 8-month-old infant with colicky abdominal pain and rectal bleeding is likely to have intussusception, which may be diagnosed on abdominal ultrasound by the presence of a 'target lesion' or by Gastrografin enema. The 'target' lesion represents the layers of the bowel, one invaginated inside the other, seen in transverse section.

Hirschsprung's disease typically presents in the first few days of life with abdominal distension, bile-stained vomiting and failure to pass meconium. The diagnosis can easily be made by the presence of a cone between collapsed distal (usually rectum) and proximal dilated bowel on a contrast enema. The cone represents the transition zone between normal proximal ganglionated bowel and distal aganglionic bowel. Confirmation of Hirschprung's disease, however, can only be made on histological biopsy.

Hypochloraemic metabolic alkalosis is typical of pyloric stenosis.

The presence of air-filled cysts in the left chest is typical of a diaphragmatic hernia, although the differential diagnosis includes congenital cystic disease of the lung. Clubbed renal calyces noted on micturating cystography will be associated with more severe vesicoureteric reflux. Dilatation of the renal pelvis without dilatation of the corresponding ureter might be due to pelviureteric junction obstruction (PUJ). Diuretic renography may distinguish an obstructed system from that of a dilated but normally draining system.

3.70 ABCD

Early closure of the fontanelles can result from primary failure of brain growth, causing microcephaly. The unfused skull bones and fontanelles allow easier passage of the fetal head during labour, and accommodate a rapidly growing brain in the first 6 months of life. Both the anterior and posterior fontanelles lie on the medial sagittal plane. Blood samples may be taken from the sagittal sinus through the anterior fontanelle in the midline. Normally, the anterior fontanelle is larger than the posterior fontanelle.

3.71 C

Cystic fibrosis may present as recurrent respiratory tract infection, for which chest physiotherapy is an important part of their management. Nasal polyps are rarely seen in children and the common cold will produce a bilateral nasal discharge. The most common cause for a unilateral nasal discharge is a foreign body, and if this has been present for some time, it will be associated with a foul smell. The discharge is often blood-stained.

3.72 ABD

Cleft lip has an increasing incidence with 1/750 affected live births. The condition is more common in males. The subsequent risk of future affected children is 5%, rising to 9% with two affected siblings. Cleft lip has an association with palate defects in up to 50% of cases.

3.73 BEF

10% of inguinal hernias in children present with irreducible hernias, the risk of which is highest in the first 3 months of life. Prompt elective surgery is essential. Simple herniotomy will suffice as the inguinal canal only develops its obliquity at the age of 11–12 years. Delivering the testicle into the wound leads to much higher complications, such as ischaemia.

3.74 BDE

Intussusception usually presents between the age of 6 months and 1 year. The most common type is an ileocolic intussusception. It is uncommon to find (<10%) a definite cause. Lymphoid hyperplasia in Peyer's patches may play a role during a viral illness. The classical history of intussusception is episodic attacks of screaming with the infant's legs being drawn up. Between these episodes the child is healthy. The child may pass 'redcurrant jelly' stools and may have a sausage-shaped abdominal mass on examination. Diagnosis can be made by ultrasound or contrast studies.

3.75 ADE

The Eustachian tube in a child is shorter and more horizontal. The opening of the auditory tube lies above the soft palate adjacent to the tubal tonsil. The bony part of the Eustachian tube perforates the petrous temporal bone.

3.76 D

Blood volume is 85 ml/kg, so a 3 kg baby would have a volume of 255 ml. The kidneys of a neonate are not mature and therefore cannot handle large sodium loads. Heat loss is of paramount importance in neonates, and theatres should be at 25 °C to prevent excessive heat loss. Due to the immature gut, parenteral nutrition is commonly used in babies following bowel operations as they cannot cope with gastric feeds. Oral feed should be given at approximately 150 ml/kg per day in the first week.

3.77 ABD

Cystic fibrosis is an autosomal recessive disease resulting from mutations in the gene located on chromosome 7. It is the most common inherited disease in white people. It typically presents in childhood, but nearly 5% are diagnosed in adults. Obstruction to the small and large intestines may occur due to the formation of a meconium ileus. Failure to secrete sodium bicarbonate or water leads to the retention of enzymes and pancreatic destruction. Other conditions associated with cystic fibrosis include chronic cholecystitis and cholelithiasis. Up to 25% of children and 45% of adults have nasal polyps. Cystic fibrosis has an association with bronchiectasis, not bronchitis.

3.78 BCD

An undescended testis is fixed to prevent progressive hypoplasia. Whilst orchidopexy does not restore full fertility, the overall incidence of fertility is improved if the testicle is brought down into the scrotum. However, fixing the testicle does not eliminate the risk of malignant change. Most testicles will descend to the normal position even if they are not within the scrotum at birth. Those that are still not in the correct position at 1 year are likely to need surgical intervention. This may be staged if the testicle cannot be brought down into the scrotum easily and without tension. Fixation of the opposite testicle is not required if it sits in the scrotum.

3.79 BCDE

Prolactin secretion is controlled by the hypothalamus through the release of dopamine, which has an inhibitory effect. There are no known hypothalamic prolactin-releasing hormones, although both TRH and VIP stimulate prolactin secretion – this is **not**, however, of physiological importance. Prolactin secretion increases after surgery, and trauma, as part of the stress response. A physiological rise in prolactin levels is seen during pregnancy and breast-feeding. Prolactin stimulates the secretion of breast milk and reduces gonadal activity. Other common causes of hyperprolactinaemia are a prolactin-secreting tumour and drugs such as dopaminergic-receptor blockers

3.80 ABCE

Exomphalos has a frequent association with other structural and chromosomal abnormalities leading to a mortality rate in the region of 25% after birth. Herniated organs in exomphalos are covered by a membrane derived from the umbilical cord and therefore the bowel and liver are not damaged by being outside the fetal abdomen. The liver is frequently herniated in exomphalos. In small exomphalos defects, a loop of bowel may herniate into the umbilical cord, thus the umbilical cord clamp may involve this loop of intestine if placed too close to the infant's abdominal wall.

3.81 BD

Pyloric stenosis presents with projectile vomiting and has a male predilection. It typically presents in the sixth week of life and there is sometimes a family history. If there has been persistent vomiting, the child may be dehydrated and have hypokalaemia and a metabolic alkalosis. A test feed with clinical examination is still widely used to identify pyloric stenosis. However, ultrasound is routinely performed and may demonstrate pyloric stenosis in up to 90% of cases.

3.82 ABCD

Abdominal pain in a 4-year-old infant can be due to a myriad of causes, many of them outside the abdomen. Intestinal atresia is not a cause of abdominal pain in a 4-year-old as it would present in the first few days of life.

3.83 BC

The incidence of UDT in term infants is 3–4%. In preterm babies the incidence is 30%. 75% of UDT descend by 1 year and most of these descend in the first 3 months. Placement in the scrotum does not change the risk of tumour development but places the testis in a palpable position. Studies have shown that spermatogenesis becomes impaired if orchidopexy is performed after 1 year. Laparoscopy is the investigation (and treatment) of choice for intra-abdominal testes.

3.84 BDE

The metabolic upset with pyloric stenosis is typically a hypokalaemic hypochloraemic metabolic alkalosis. Although the metabolic disturbance is quite typical, the diagnosis should be made on clinical grounds and blood samples monitored to assess resuscitation. A test feed is usually used to aid diagnosis. Ultrasound is now used routinely for investigation. Males are more frequently affected than females. Jaundice is an association in about 10% of children with pyloric stenosis.

3.85 BD

Inguinal hernia occurring in infancy is usually of the indirect variety and is due to the presence of a widely patent processus vaginalis into which bowel or ovary may herniate. The processus vaginalis normally obliterates at about 40 weeks' gestation. Therefore, inguinal hernia is more common in infants born prematurely. The risk of strangulation is approximately 1 in 3. Waiting until an infant is about 10 kg in weight (approximately 1 year of age) places a significant number of infants at risk of bowel, testicular or ovarian damage. Infants with inguinal hernia require a simple herniotomy (ligation of hernial sac) and not a herniorrhaphy.

3.86 CD

Premature infants do not always require ventilation in the first 24 hours after birth. Premature infants have a much higher insensible fluid loss than adults, because of the thinner skin and greater body surface area to weight ratio. This means that careful attention must be paid to the environment in which these infants are cared for. When infants require long-term venous access, it is occasionally necessary to operatively insert a central line into the internal jugular vein. Premature infants are at a high risk of developing necrotising enterocolitis. Pyloric stenosis is known to occur in premature infants.

3.87 ABCE

Hirschsprung's disease is a congenital abnormality characterised by the absence of ganglion cells in the myenteric plexus of the autonomic nervous system. The disease almost always involves the rectum and spreads for a variable distance proximally. In rare instances, it can involve the entire intestine. Presentation in the adult is well described. It also has an association with Down's syndrome. Hirschsprung's disease is treated by resection of the aganglionic segment and coloanal reconstruction (a 'pull-through' procedure).

3.88 ADE

Intussusception, is the commonest cause of small bowel obstruction in a child under the age of 18 months. The classical presentation is of colicky abdominal pain associated with 'redcurrant jelly' stools rather than the 'brick-red' coloured stool. The latter is more typical of a bleeding Meckel's diverticulum. A lead-point occurs in over 25% of children presenting over the age of 18 months with an intussusception. A pathological lead-point is less common under this age. Approximately 75% of children with an intussusception can be treated effectively with an air enema, in which oxygen is gently pumped into an infant's rectum to 'blow' the intussusception back. An air enema should not be attempted in a child with peritonitis or continuing signs of shock despite appropriate resuscitation – emergency surgery should not be delayed in these cases.

3.89 ACDE

Oesophageal atresia is a complex congenital abnormality which is frequently associated with other structural abnormalities including vertebral, cardiac, renal and limb abnormalities. Oesophageal atresia can occur without a tracheo-oesophageal fistula. When there is a long gap between the upper and lower pouches (greater than approximately four vertebral bodies) definitive reconstruction of the oesophagus may be delayed until the child is over 1 year of age. Maternal polyhydramnios is a feature of oesophageal atresia.

3.90 ABD

Diaphragmatic hernia usually occurs due to failure of closure of the pleuroperitoneal canal (8th week). It is associated with hypoplasia of the lungs and may present with respiratory distress at birth. 85% of congenital diaphragmatic hernias are left-sided and over 50% are associated with congenital defects. Surgical correction is delayed until the infant is stable. Infants may require inotropic support and pulmonary vasodilators (e.g. nitric oxide) or extracorporeal membrane oxygenation. Late presentations include vomiting and a failure to thrive.

3.91 A

Duodenal atresia is more frequent in children with Down's syndrome (trisomy 21). Surgery to correct duodenal atresia usually involves a duodenostomy, which may be delayed for 3 or 4 days after birth. The typical X-ray appearance of a double-bubble is usually quite obvious when the child is a few hours old.

3.92 ABE

A hydrocele in an infant is due to a persistent patent processus vaginalis, which allows fluid to communicate between the abdomen and scrotum. The processus vaginalis may continue to obliterate in the first 12 months of a child's life, and the child can be observed until after this age. Repair is necessary if the hydrocele persists, or presents de novo. Hydroceles may also occur in females. Surgery involves simple division of the patent processus vaginalis. When the patent processus vaginalis does not extend as far as the testicle, the hydrocele fluid may not surround the testicle.

3.93 ABD

A mal-descended testis is one which has failed to reach the normal low position in the scrotum. Maldescent can be either arrested descent (cryptorchidism), where the testis is found at some point along the line of normal descent (intra-abdominal, inguinal canal, superficial inguinal pouch or high scrotum), or less commonly in a position not on the normal line of descent, i.e. ectopic: penile, superficial inguinal or femoral.

3.94 CD

A hydrocele developing in this age group is usually due to a patent processus vaginalis at or near the deep inguinal ring, and so repair of hydrocele should be directed at the cause. A groin incision is made to obliterate the patent processus. Aspiration serves no purpose and will lead to inevitable recurrence. Resolution is also unlikely, as the processus will not close spontaneously. These cases are ideal for day surgery.

ANSWERS – CHAPTER 4: ABDOMEN

4.1 AD

The ischiorectal fossae, more accurately termed the 'ischioanal fossae', are wedge-shaped, fascia-lined spaces between the perianal skin and levator ani. The levator ani group is a thin muscular sheet with four groups of fibres: levator prostatae (men) or sphincter vaginae (women); puborectalis; pubococcygeus; and iliococcygeus. This group of muscles is supplied by S2–S4 roots. The levator ani also originates from the body of the pubis and the ischial spine. Whereas the aorta bifurcates at L4, the levator ani is found around the coccygeal level.

4.2 Surface/radiological anatomy of the anterior abdominal wall

1. B L4 vertebral body
2. F Sacroiliac joint
3. D Mid-inguinal point
4. J 12th rib

The aorta divides at the level of the L4 vertebral body, to the left and anterior to the inferior vena cava. It is imprecise to state that it divides at the level of the umbilicus, as this is a variable surface anatomical landmark, which is lower in obese people.

The ureter crosses the pelvic brim at the sacroiliac joint.

The femoral artery passes under the inguinal ligament at the mid-inguinal point.

The upper pole of the kidney lies on the 12th rib, on each side.

4.3 ABC

The superior mesenteric artery (SMA) supplies the entire small intestine except the proximal duodenum. The SMA also supplies the caecum, ascending colon and half the transverse colon. The origin of the SMA lies behind the neck of the pancreas (at level L1). The SMA passes forward and downward in front of the uncinate process and the third part of the duodenum. Throughout, the superior mesenteric vein lies to its right. The splenic vein grooves the posterosuperior aspect of the pancreas and passes above the SMA.

4.4 ABCD

The epiploic foramen (of Winslow) is the communicating cavity between the greater and lesser sacs. It is an important surgical area, particularly for open cholecystectomy and gastrectomy. The lower boundary of the foramen is formed by the first part of the duodenum. The caudate lobe is the only part of the liver present in the lesser sac. It also forms the roof of the epiploic foramen. In the free edge of the lesser sac run the hepatic artery, portal vein and common bile duct.

4.5 AB

Hesselbach's triangle is the thin and weak part of the posterior wall of the inguinal canal covered only by transversalis fascia and peritoneum, through which direct inguinal hernias arise. Its borders are the inferior epigastric artery, the inguinal ligament and the lateral border of the rectus abdominis muscle.

4.6 CDE

The epiploic foramen (of Winslow) is the communicating cavity between the greater and lesser sacs. The caudate lobe of the liver forms the superior boundary. Anteriorly is the free border of the lesser omentum: its two layers containing the hepatic artery, common bile duct and portal vein. Posteriorly is the IVC, covered by peritoneum. Inferiorly is the first part of the duodenum (covered by peritoneum) and the hepatic artery. The gastroduodenal artery lies virtually anterior to the portal vein and is thus anterior to the epiploic foramen. In Pringle's manoeuvre pressure is applied to the free edge of the lesser sac. This temporary manoeuvre is used to control major bleeding from a lacerated liver. The portal vein lies anterior to the common bile duct and the hepatic artery in this free edge.

4.7 AC

The psoas muscle has an origin from the transverse processes, bodies and intervertebral discs of T12–L5 and inserts along with the iliacus into the lesser trochanter. It is innervated by the lumbar plexus (L2–L4). The iliacus is supplied by the femoral nerve.

4.8 Anatomy of abdominal vasculature

1. **C Left gastric vein**
2. **F Gastroduodenal artery**
3. **A Inferior mesenteric vein**
4. **D Right renal artery**

The left gastric vein is continuous with the hemiazygos system (systemic) through the oesophageal branches and with the portal vein.
The gastroduodenal artery is liable to erosion from duodenal ulcers as it lies behind the first part of the duodenum. This can cause a profuse upper GI bleed.
The inferior mesenteric vein drains into the splenic vein.
The right renal artery lies posterior to the inferior vena cava (whereas the common iliac veins lie posterior to the arteries).

4.9 ABE

The body of the uterus is related anteriorly to the superior surface of the bladder or coils of small bowel. Posteriorly lies the pouch of Douglas. The body of the uterus is covered with peritoneum except where it is reflected off the bladder and at the broad ligaments. The uterine artery arises from the internal iliac artery and runs in the base of the broad ligament. The nerves of the uterus are derived from the inferior hypogastric plexus.

4.10 DE

The liver is mostly covered by peritoneum except for the bare area which lies to the right of the IVC between the coronary ligaments. The liver may be divided into 8 anatomical segments. The right suprarenal gland (but not the left), kidney,right colic flexure, the duodenum and the gallbladder are in contact with the liver. The falciform ligament connects the liver to the anterior abdominal wall. The liver is largely separated from the diaphragm by the subphrenic recesses of the peritoneal cavity.

4.11 Anatomy of the viscera and organs in the abdomen

1. H Kidney
2. B Ileum
3. G Meckel's diverticulum
4. F Pancreas
5. D Stomach

The left kidney has the inferior mesenteric vein passing over its anterior medial border.

The root of the mesentery of the small bowel is attached below to the brim of the pelvis over the left sacroiliac joint.

Meckel's diverticulum is frequently attached to the umbilicus either directly or indirectly by a fibrous band.

The tail of the pancreas lies in the lienorenal ligament touching the hilum of the spleen.

The left gastric vein forms portosystemic anastomoses through its ascending oesophageal branches with the hemiazygos system.

4.12 ABE

The territory of the mesenteric veins essentially follows that of their arteries. The inferior mesenteric vein drains the rectum via the superior rectal vein. The inferior mesenteric vein lies superficially, immediately below the peritoneum and to the left of the inferior mesenteric artery. After crossing over the left renal vein and under the body of the pancreas, it joins the splenic vein (the portal vein is formed downstream by the confluence of the splenic vein and superior mesenteric vein), though variations occur. Thus, the superior mesenteric and splenic veins are considered tributaries of the portal vein, whereas the inferior mesenteric vein is not. The ileum is drained by the superior mesenteric vein as it is part of the mid-gut.

4.13 BDE

The portal vein is the confluence of the superior mesenteric vein after its union with the splenic vein. It lies in front of the IVC, and passes upwards behind the neck of the pancreas and first part of the duodenum. It runs in the free edge of the lesser omentum, forming the anterior boundary of the epiploic foramen. The portal vein receives tributaries from the left and right gastric, cystic and superior pancreaticoduodenal veins.

4.14 AB

As soon as the aorta passes below the aortic hiatus, it gives off the coeliac plexus (T12). The plexus has three direct branches: left gastric, hepatic and splenic (mnemonic: **l**eft-**h**and **s**ide). The right gastric and gastroduodenal arteries are branches of the hepatic artery. The superior pancreatico-duodenal artery is a branch of the gastroduodenal artery.

4.15 ABD

Both renal veins drain directly into the IVC. The left renal vein has further to travel and is thus longer. The right suprarenal gland and right gonad have veins that drain directly into the IVC. The left suprarenal gland and left gonad drain into the left renal vein first. The IVC possesses a variable non-functioning valve at its orifice into the right atrium.

4.16 All true

Portal vein thrombosis may occur secondarily to thrombophilia or septic thrombophlebitis, possibly in severe appendicitis. It is one of the causes of small bowel infarction. It may result in portal hypertension with small intestinal varices and splenomegaly.

4.17 BCDE

The sigmoid colon is supplied by the sigmoid branches of the inferior mesenteric artery. Sacral radicular branches are given off by the lateral sacral arteries and feed into the anterior and posterior spinal vessels of the sacral segments of the spinal cord. Both the trochanteric and cruciate anastomoses are fed by descending branches of the superior and inferior gluteal arteries, whilst the iliolumbar and superior gluteal arteries contribute to the anterior superior iliac spine anastomosis. The anterior division of the internal iliac artery supplies the bladder.

4.18 AD

Scrotal skin drains to the inguinal lymph nodes as does the distal end of the anal canal. The uterus drains mainly to the external iliac nodes but it is also possible for lymph to reach the inguinal nodes via the round ligament and inguinal canal. While lymph from the body of the uterus may reach the inguinal nodes, the cervix does not drain to the inguinal lymph nodes but to the external and internal iliac nodes that run in front of or behind the ureter. The cervix also drains to the sacral nodes via the uterosacral ligaments. The testes and fallopian tubes drain to the para-aortic nodes via lymphatics running back with the gonadal arteries.

4.19 ABCE

The superficial inguinal lymph nodes comprise a proximal group, below the inguinal ligament, and a distal group, lying alongside the termination of the great saphenous vein. The lateral nodes of the former group drain the buttock and back, and also the flank below the waist. The medial nodes drain the anterior abdominal wall below the umbilicus, including the external genitalia (excluding the testis), lower anal canal and perineum. The testes drain to the para-aortic nodes via lymphatics running back with the gonadal arteries. The fundus of the uterus drains via lymphatics accompanying the round ligament. The distal group of nodes drain superficial lymphatics from the lower limb.

4.20 Anatomy of the posterior abdominal wall

1. B Psoas major muscle
2. D Ureter
3. E Sympathetic trunk
4. F Ilioinguinal nerve

A psoas abscess tracts within the tough psoas fascia to point below the inguinal ligament in the femoral triangle.
The left ureter crosses the pelvic brim over the sacroiliac joint in front of the divisions of the common iliac vessels within the apex of the V-shaped root of the sigmoid mesentery.
The left sympathetic trunk lies behind the left margin of the aorta.
The ilioinguinal nerve lies behind the kidney on each side.

4.21 AB

Femoral hernias have a high risk of strangulation owing to the usually narrow femoral canal and hernial neck. The hernia itself is usually small and easily missed in obese people. They are more common in females. The neck of the sac lies below the level of the inguinal ligament, but if large, the hernial sac itself will extend anterior and above it. Scrotal skin invagination will reveal an empty inguinal canal.

4.22 DEF

Most patients with gallstones are asymptomatic. The pain of biliary colic is due to gallbladder distension resulting from temporary cystic duct obstruction from a calculus impacted in Hartmann's pouch. Symptoms are relieved following spontaneous disimpaction. A mucocele is a gallbladder distended with mucus, which is not normally infected. An empyema is an intraluminal abscess whereby the gallbladder wall remains intact. Though it can lead to major sepsis, it is usually associated with lesser degrees of systemic disturbance. Acute cholecystitis infrequently progresses to perforation, but if it occurs it is usually at the fundus, or occasionally adjacent to an impacted stone.

4.23 AB

Bright-red rectal bleeding and excessive passage of mucus are present in >90% of cases of solitary rectal ulcer syndrome. The condition itself is felt to be related to rectal trauma created by varying degrees of rectal prolapse, though some believe it to be partly due to self-digitation. Histological features are those of smooth muscle fibres extending from a thickened muscularis mucosa into the lamina propria with associated fibrosis and mucosal ulceration. Palisading basal cells are a feature of basal-cell carcinoma. Solitary rectal ulcer syndrome has a very high recurrence rate following simple excision of visible rectal lesions. It is a very difficult condition to treat, though biofeedback may be of benefit. Rectopexy has been attempted in those who do not respond, with universally poor results. Patients not infrequently come to stoma formation.

4.24 BCD

Indications for surgery in patients with ulcerative colitis may include: in acute cases, a failure to respond after 5 days of optimal medical treatment; acute toxic megacolon with or without perforation; perforation; severe bleeding; failure of adequate medical treatment for chronic disease over a prolonged period; and the presence of confirmed dysplasia of any severity on colonic biopsies. Total colitis increases the long-term risk of developing colorectal carcinoma, but is not in itself an indication for surgery.

4.25 D

Superior mesenteric artery emboli are responsible for between 40 and 50% of episodes of acute mesenteric ischaemia. They usually originate from a mural or atrial thrombus. Superior mesenteric artery embolus tends to lodge at points of normal anatomical narrowings just distal to the origin of the major branch. The surgical options must be balanced against the quality of life that may be expected if the operation succeeds. In the USA, an aggressive policy is carried out using arterial embolectomy and revascularisation procedures if the bowel is potentially viable. The option of extensive resection followed by TPN can be considered in a younger patient, but closure of the abdomen and effective pain control is likely to be more appropriate in elderly patients.

4.26 Abdominal disease
1. C Mesenteric ischaemia
2. D Crohn's disease
3. F Appendix mass
The finding of atrial fibrillation in a patient with sudden-onset abdominal pain must raise the possibility of an embolic event. Embolism accounts for 25–30% of patients with mesenteric ischaemia. It is notoriously difficult to diagnose and the passage of blood per rectum is relatively rare.
A longer history of diarrhoea and vomiting over several months, together with a vague right iliac fossa mass and established microcytic anaemia, is more suggestive of Crohn's disease, due to iron loss from haemorrhage. A macrocytic anaemia may also be seen as a result of vitamin B_{12} malabsorption due to terminal ileitis.
An appendix mass forms when an inflamed appendix perforates locally and pus is prevented from spreading throughout the peritoneal cavity by adherent omentum and small bowel. The patient has a history suggesting appendicitis, and occasionally a tender mass may be felt in the right iliac fossa.

4.27 ACDE
Complications of laparoscopic surgery are usually related to Verres needle insertion and insufflation, i.e. abdominal wall emphysema, trocar injuries to the bowel, bladder or major vessels. Diathermy or laser injuries usually occur off-screen but may also be directly on-screen. Pneumothorax, carbon dioxide embolus and deep vein thrombosis are the other well-known complications.

4.28 ABD
Risk factors for colorectal carcinoma include ulcerative colitis, familial adenomatous polyposis and Gardner's syndrome. These patients should be screened on a regular basis. Peutz–Jeghers' syndrome is an autosomal dominant condition characterised by circumoral mucocutaneous pigmentation associated with hamartomas in the small bowel. Hamartomas have been described in the stomach and colon. These polyps are multiple and present in childhood with bleeding, anaemia or small bowel obstruction.

4.29 C

Crohn's disease runs a chronic relapsing course and cannot be cured by surgical excision. Bowel should be resected back to macroscopically normal intestine. When there are several, short-segment, small bowel strictures, then multiple stricturoplasties are preferred to multiple small bowel resections, as the emphasis is on preservation of small bowel length. If proctocolectomy is indicated, an intersphincteric dissection should be performed to preserve perirectal tissues and aid postoperative wound closure. Perianal abscesses, as at other times, require surgical drainage, but the surgery should be conservative. Antibiotics (e.g. metronidazole, ciprofloxacin) are helpful in controlling many of the anal manifestations of Crohn's disease.

4.30 BCE

Colorectal cancer is the second commonest malignant cause of death in the UK after lung cancer. There is a marked male predominance for rectal cancer. The incidence is much less in Africa and Asia than in Western countries, perhaps reflecting diet and other environmental factors. There is an increasing relative incidence of right-sided to left-sided colonic carcinoma in Western countries. 30% of patients with colorectal cancer have hepatic metastases and 10% have pulmonary metastases at time of presentation.

4.31 DE

Early poor prognostic factors for acute pancreatitis include: a blood glucose level of >11 mmol/l in the absence of previously diagnosed diabetes; a serum calcium concentration of <2 mmol/l; a WCC $>15 \times 10^9$/l; pO_2 <8 kPa; a blood urea concentration of >16 mmol/l despite adequate fluid replacement; serum albumin level of <32 g/l; serum AST (SGOT) >200 U/l; and serum LDH >600 IU/l. These criteria are based on Ranson and Imrie systems. Haemoglobin and the degree of elevation of serum amylase are not predictors of outcome. C-reactive protein is also a good independent prognostic indicator.

4.32 Abdominal pain investigations

1. **A FBC**
2. **C Erect CXR**
3. **F Mesenteric angiography**
4. **D Supine AXR**

The most likely diagnosis for the first patient is appendicitis – a clinical diagnosis. FBC measurement is useful in lending support to the diagnosis, in that it may show a neutrophilia, but a normal reading should not affect management. No other investigations listed are relevant.

Patient 2 has a good history for perforation of a viscus, probably a peptic ulcer – she is on several ulcer-promoting medications. An erect CXR should be performed after the patient has been upright for several minutes to look for free gas under the diaphragm.

Whilst an FBC is important in patient 3 it will not lead to diagnosing the cause of the problem. A mesenteric angiogram is useful if the patient is bleeding at a rate of >1 ml/min.

Patient 4 may be developing acute intestinal obstruction. This is more likely after operations on the lower part of the abdomen. A supine AXR will aim to show any dilated loops.

4.33 ACD

Typical endoscopic features of Crohn's disease include: mucosal erythema; aphthous ulceration; loss of the normal vascular pattern; mucosal oedema; and deep fissuring ulceration with a cobblestone appearance. Microadenomas are associated with FAP. Pseudomembranes are endoscopic features of pseudomembranous colitis.

4.34 ABE

Typical radiological features of acute ulcerative colitis on plain AXR include: loss of the haustral fold pattern; mucosal irregularity or ulceration; tubular shaped colon (lead-pipe appearance); and absence of faecal residue within the actively inflamed part of the colon. Left-sided faecal loading is common in constipated patients. The 'beak sign' is seen on an instant enema in sigmoid volvulus.

4.35 ABCE

The most prominent cutaneous manifestation of carcinoid syndrome is paroxysmal flushing (occurs in 75% of patients). It generally affects the face and central trunk. Flushing may be precipitated or exacerbated by hot food, chocolate, alcohol, cheese and stress. Systemic symptoms preceding or accompanying paroxysmal flushing include: abdominal pain, diarrhoea, bronchospasm, hypotension and wheezing. Although the tumours are frequently unresectable, debulking has been shown to provide palliative relief. Symptoms may also be improved by octreotide (somatostatin analogue).

4.36 BCD

Endoscopic visual appearances alone sometimes allow one to differentiate between ulcerative colitis and Crohn's disease, but there is a large overlap in macroscopic findings. Definitive diagnosis requires histology, but even with histology the diagnosis is indeterminate in 10–15% of cases. An 'instant' enema is performed without bowel preparation. It is helpful if the anatomical extent of disease needs to be determined at initial presentation in order to guide appropriate management. Colonoscopy should only be performed when the disease is mildly active. A proximal colonic stool on plain AXR in a patient with ulcerative colitis suggests that the proximal large bowel is not significantly inflamed.

4.37 D

The incidence of invasive cancer in colorectal polyps depends on both the polyp size and polyp type. Overall, the incidence in polyps of <1 cm is approximately 1%, in polyps 1–2 cm is approximately 10% and in polyps >2 cm is approximately 50%. Polyps in the rectum have a higher risk of malignancy than elsewhere in the colon. Villous adenomas have a greater risk of malignant change than tubular adenomas of the same size. According to the 'adenoma–carcinoma sequence', the majority of colorectal carcinomas arise in adenomatous polyps, but only a small proportion of polyps will become malignant.

4.38 ACD

Epigastric hernias are multiple in about 30% of cases, and usually contain extraperitoneal fat, although they can sometimes contain small bowel. They are frequently irreducible, but are often more easily seen than felt. Usually small, they are repaired by excision of the extraperitoneal fat and sac, and a Mayo-type repair. Meshed repair is rarely required, but should be considered if the defect is large and the surrounding tissues are lax.

4.39 ABCE

Dermatomyositis has a 25% association with malignancy. The earliest cutaneous finding is oedema and erythema of the eyelids, causing a colour change (pinkish purple) and termed a 'heliotrope rash'. The most common malignancies associated with dermatomyositis are carcinoma of the ovary, breast, lung, cervix and GI tract. Dermatomyositis has been reported to precede development of the neoplasm by 5 years. Treatment of the malignancy results in improvement of the cutaneous changes.

4.40 ADE

Although acute acalculous cholecystitis can arise spontaneously, it is especially common in ITU patients following major trauma, surgery or sepsis. It is thought to be related to bile stasis. Factors contributing to increased bile viscosity include pyrexia and dehydration. Diagnosis is initially made by suspicion of those patients at risk, and the subsequent findings of gallbladder wall-thickening and pericholecystic fluid on ultrasound in the absence of gallstones. In acute cholecystitis 90% of cases are due to gallstones.

4.41 ABE

The approximate incidences of involvement are: ileocaecal regions only, 40%; colon only, 25%; ileum only, 25%; extensive small bowel disease, 5%; and miscellaneous (e.g. confined to the anorectum, oral, gastric regions), 2%.

4.42 ABCE

Various methods have been used to help preserve the spleen. Omental patch repair is helpful in allowing additional support for sutures that would otherwise cut out and exacerbate bleeding. Topical thrombogenic agents may be used including gelatine, gelatine sponge, fibrin glue and collagen. Induced hypotension is never used and may seriously risk life in an already haemorrhaging patient. Partial splenectomy is useful when damage is localised. Other techniques include direct suture repair using atraumatic needles, or mattress sutures with Teflon buttresses, or using an argon-beam laser.

4.43 AE

The Child–Pugh classification of hepatocellular function in cirrhosis includes details of serum bilirubin, serum albumin, the presence of ascites, encephalopathy and the prothrombin time. Patients are scored into groups A, B or C, with increasing mortality risk from surgery.

4.44 AC

Bile-stained vomiting is a serious sign in any child and surgical causes need to be considered. Bile-stained vomiting occurs when the cause of the obstruction is distal to the ampulla of Vater. This is the case with both mid-gut volvulus (obstruction is in the third part of the duodenum) and intussusception. In pyloric stenosis and gastro-oesophageal reflux, the vomit is generally of altered feed; the 'vomiting' of oesophageal atresia is that of unaltered milk.

4.45 D

Gallstone ileus follows spontaneous perforation of the gallbladder into the duodenum. Offending calculi, generally a single stone, usually impact in the distal ileum just proximal to the ileocaecal junction, which is the narrowest part of the small bowel. Obstruction is usually incomplete, making a preoperative diagnosis difficult. Dilated small bowel loops and aerobilia may be seen on AXR, but the obstructing calculus is only occasionally seen (10%).

4.46 CDE

The extent of distal intramural spread of rectal cancer is usually <1 cm, so that a distal clearance of 2 cm is considered an adequate clearance margin for the majority of rectal cancers. The mesorectum contains an abundance of lymphatic and vascular channels. Irrigation of the divided bowel ends with cytotoxic solutions (such as chlorhexidine or iodine) reduces local tumour recurrence in uncontrolled series. However, there are no randomised controlled trials to date.

4.47 Abdominal pain investigations – diagnostic

1. B Serum amylase
2. H Barium meal – small bowel follow-through
3. C Erect CXR
4. A FBC

Serum amylase estimation would be the most appropriate investigation for the first clinical case scenario, as the most likely diagnosis is pancreatitis. A subsequent CT may be needed if findings are equivocal.

The history of the young man is suggestive of Crohn's disease and a barium meal with small bowel follow-through would be the most appropriate.

The third patient is most likely to have a perforated peptic ulcer as evidenced by the epigastric pain, shallow respirations and tachycardia. This would be suspected because of her oral steroid and non-steroidal intake. An erect CXR would be the most appropriate investigation.

The most appropriate investigation in the fourth patient would be a full blood count as the rectal bleeding has led her to become tachycardic and hypotensive. If she continues to bleed profusely, she will require a mesenteric angiogram and possible embolisation of the bleeding vessel.

4.48 ACD

Most patients who undergo a gastrectomy fail to regain their preoperative weight. Low serum calcium, vitamin C and iron levels (but not frank deficiency) are seen, as the hypochlorhydria interferes with their absorption. Vitamin B_{12} deficiency develops due to diminished levels of intrinsic factor from the stomach. This may be corrected by injections of hydroxocobalamin every 3 months.

4.49 BCDE

In adults, full-thickness rectal prolapse is seen predominantly in females. Rectal prolapse most commonly occurs in very young or elderly people. Faecal incontinence may be a presenting feature, but a prolapsing mass is most commonly described. Surgical treatment is complex, as numerous operations have been variably described. The prolapse may be repaired via perineal (e.g. Delorme's or Altmeier's procedures, or recto-sigmoidectomy) or abdominal approaches. The latter may be open or laparoscopic and involve mobilising the rectum and suturing to the sacral promontory or partially wrapping the rectum in a mesh (Ripstein's procedure). The overall success of these approaches is often disappointing as the condition is still poorly understood and the surgical procedures do not appear to address the underlying problem.

4.50 ACDE

Carcinoid tumours are neuroendocrine in origin. They commonly occur in the small bowel and 85% of appendix neoplasms are known to be carcinoid in origin. Carcinoid tumours can also occur in extraintestinal sites such as the bronchus. A small proportion of patients with carcinoid tumours develop the carcinoid syndrome (flushing, bronchospasm and diarrhoea due to the secretion of 5-hydroxytryptamine [5-HT, serotonin], bradykinin and histamine).

4.51 ABC

Several series show a 25–30% 5-year survival rate following resection of hepatic metastases from colorectal cancer in the absence of other metastatic or recurrent disease. The best surgical results are achieved by resection along hepatic segmental lines. Although chemotherapy often slows or regresses tumour growth, it is not curative. Liver metastases are present in about 25% of patients at the time of diagnosis of the primary tumour. These lesions are relatively radioresistant.

4.52 CDE

Colorectal cancer is inherited in only 10% of cases. Both metachronous and synchronous cancers occur in 5% of cases. Colorectal cancer is inevitable in cases of untreated FAP, with an average age of presentation in the third decade. The cumulative lifetime risk approaches 100%. Of all prognostic factors for colorectal cancer, the clinical stage of disease is the most important.

4.53 B

Barium enema is less sensitive than colonoscopy for the assessment of polyps as it may miss smaller <1 cm polyps. However, barium enema is more sensitive for the assessment of diverticular disease than colonoscopy, and is more able to demonstrate the extent and pattern of disease. CT is the modality of choice for the evaluation of acute diverticulitis as it can demonstrate the extent of disease and associated complications, e.g. abscess collections. Collagenous colitis is a histological diagnosis and requires colonic biopsies. The imaging and endoscopic appearances of the bowel are normal in collagenous colitis. Double-contrast studies (barium and air) provide greater mucosal detail and are superior to single-contrast studies. Barium enema, though often demonstrating the appendiceal lumen, is not used for the assessment of appendiceal pathology.

4.54 Acid–base balance

		pH	$PaCO_2$	HCO_3^-
1.	A	7.20	3.1	11
2.	C	7.56	3.0	30
3.	B	7.42	6.1	35

Intestinal obstruction would lead to loss of fluid from the intravascular space and produce third-space loss. The presence of peritonitis and a grossly elevated WBC strongly suggest the presence of infarcted bowel. All these factors would produce a metabolic acidosis.

The history in the second case is suggestive of pulmonary emboli. Pulmonary emboli may occur at any stage after surgery, but most frequently after 5 days, and should be suspected in all cases of dyspnoea (earliest sign). The ensuing hyperventilation would reduce pCO_2, shifting the Henderson–Hasselbach equation to the right (reducing H^+), causing a respiratory alkalosis.

Patient 3 may not be taking deep-enough breaths due to pain from his laparotomy, which would be exacerbated by COPD from his smoking. He will therefore have a respiratory acidosis due to retained carbon dioxide. Note there is a compensatory rise in the serum bicarbonate level.

Normal values:

pH	7.35–7.45
PaO_2	>10.6 kPa
$PaCO_2$	4.7–6.0 kPa
HCO_3^-	24–30 mmol/l

4.55 ABC

Pancreatic carcinoma is more common in men and rarely develops before the age of 50 years. Cigarette smoking is 2–3 times more common in patients with pancreatic carcinoma. Pancreatic cancer has a poor outcome following chemotheraphy. A large case-control study has correlated chronic pancreatitis with an increased risk of pancreatic cancer. More than 90% of pancreatic cancers are ductal adenocarcinomas. Pain and weight loss are present in more than 75% of patients. Infrequent presentations include: glucose intolerance, palpable gallbladder, migratory thrombophlebitis and splenomegaly.

4.56 A

The appendix opens on the posteromedial wall of the caecum, lies lateral to the right ureter and right gonadal vessels and has a continuous longitudinal muscular coat. The mesoappendix carries the appendicular artery. Two small folds of peritoneum should not be confused with the mesoappendix. One extends from the front of the mesoappendix to the ileum, the ileocaecal fold (bloodless fold of Treves). The other extends from the terminal part of the root of the small bowel mesentery to the anterior wall of the caecum, the vascular fold of the caecum, containing the anterior caecal artery.

4.57 AB

Insulin affects many organs and intracellular pathways. Insulin is synthesised by the β-islet cells of the pancreas and is an anabolic hormone. It stimulates glucose storage but inhibits glucose production. In addition, it enhances protein synthesis and inhibits proteolysis. The uptake of glucose by the brain is independent of insulin.

4.58 BC

The classical radiological features of Crohn's disease on small bowel imaging include: mucosal ulceration; fissuring (rose-thorn ulcers); thickening of the valvulae conniventes; fistulas to other intraperitoneal viscera or skin; luminal narrowing (with or without prestenotic dilatation); bowel wall oedema (thickening); and skip lesions. Intramural cysts are a feature of pneumatosis coli. Patients with Crohn's disease may also have a shortened small bowel as a result of previous resections.

4.59 ABC

The ascending and transverse colon are involved in the regulation of intraluminal fluid volume as well as sodium and water absorption. The left colon is the site for final modulation of intraluminal contents before evacuation. More than 90% of short-chain fatty acids are taken up by colonic mucosal cells. Chloride absorption occurs by a passive energy-independent mechanism, being absorbed together with sodium. Bicarbonate is secreted by the colon, by an energy-requiring process. Bile salts are absorbed in the terminal ileum.

4.60 D

Diverticula occur between the mesenteric and the antimesenteric taeniae. The diverticula are of the pulsion type and consist of outpouchings of mucosa that have herniated through the circular muscle. The circular muscle of affected bowel is thickened, resulting in shortening. Asians have an increased incidence of right-sided colonic diverticular disease, and this tends to occur in younger patients than left-sided disease.

4.61 Acid–base balance

1. D Respiratory acidosis

2. A Metabolic acidosis

3. E Respiratory alkalosis

Patients who suffer from chronic obstructive pulmonary disease usually have a respiratory acidosis with a compensatory metabolic alkalosis. In cases where there is an infective exacerbation, respiratory acidosis becomes the predominant feature with marked CO_2 retention.

A serum amylase level of four times the normal value is pathognomic of pancreatitis. Patients with severe acute pancreatitis will usually be acidotic from a number of causes: hypovolaemic shock, acute renal failure and lactic acidosis.

The third case is indicative of a pulmonary embolism. The first indication of a PE is dyspnoea. The patient will be hyperventilating, so producing a respiratory alkalosis. Following a lobectomy, the blood gas analysis should not be grossly altered and a normal pH should be seen.

4.62 BE

The terminal ileum is the primary site for absorption of the fat-soluble vitamins B_{12} and K. In addition, bile salts are predominantly absorbed here. Calcium and folic acid are mainly absorbed in the jejunum.

4.63 ACD

One of the functions of the spleen is the sequestration and phagocytosis of old or abnormal red cells. Therefore, in a postsplenectomy patient, red-cell inclusion bodies may be present producing target cells, Howell–Jolly bodies and sideroblasts. Punctate basophilia is seen in patients with lead poisoning, thalassaemia and haemolytic anaemia due to pyrimidine-5-nucleotidase deficiency. Rouleaux formation is the tendency for red cells to stack up like a pile of coins. The amount of rouleaux formation is determined by the concentration of protein in the plasma.

4.64 AB

Rectal bleeding is the most common initial symptom (45% of cases). 30% of patients complain of pain or sensation of a mass. The human papillomavirus (usually type 16) may cause intraepithelial neoplasia, which with time progresses to anal carcinoma. This virus is found in approximately 70% of patients. Other risk factors for anal carcinoma include a history of cervical or vaginal cancer, history of sexually transmitted disease and immunosuppression following solid organ transplantation. Lymphatic drainage – above the dentate line flows to the perirectal and paravertebral nodes; below the dentate line, drainage is through the inguinal and femoral nodes. Anal carcinoma is relatively radiosensitive. Presently, combination radiotherapy and chemotherapy (5-FU ± mitomycin or 5-FU and cisplatin) is used as initial standard, first-line treatment. Abdominoperineal resection is reserved for recurrent or resistant tumours.

4.65 ACE

Pseudomembranous colitis (PMC) has been reported to occur following the use of a wide range of antibiotics. A single dose of antibiotic may be enough to cause PMC. The clinical effects are due to *Clostridium difficile* toxin, which may be isolated in the stool in over 90% of affected patients. *Clostridium difficile* itself is difficult to culture under normal circumstances. Typically, yellow plaques form on the mucosal surface and comprise epithelial debris, mucin, fibrin and polymorphs. The treatment of choice is oral metronidazole or vancomycin. The condition uncommonly progresses to toxic megacolon and perforation.

4.66 BCEF

Ocular extraintestinal manifestations of IBD include episcleritis and uveitis. Cutaneous manifestations include erythema nodosum and pyoderma gangrenosum. 75% of patients with primary sclerosing cholangitis have underlying ulcerative colitis. Sclerosing cholangitis rarely occurs with Crohn's disease. Hepatic cirrhosis occurs in 1–5% of patients with ulcerative colitis, and only rarely with Crohn's. Other hepatobiliary manifestations include mild abnormalities of liver function tests, fatty liver, pericholangitis and bile duct carcinoma. Ankylosing spondylitis occurs in 5% of cases of IBD. Arthritis (large joint) is the most common extraintestinal manifestation of IBD. Urinary calculi form in up to 10% of IBD patients, especially those with an ileostomy.

4.67 CE

Abdominal signs may be masked by steroids. Toxic dilatation is more common in patients with ulcerative colitis than with Crohn's disease. Sequential AXR is an important means of monitoring the development of toxic dilatation in patients with total severe colitis. A colonic diameter of >6.5 cm in an unwell patient indicates the presence of toxic megacolon. A diameter of this size in a well patient without abdominal signs is unlikely to be due to toxic dilatation. In severe ulcerative colitis, the haemoglobin and serum albumin levels fall, whereas the WBC, ESR and CRP are elevated. Growth retardation is a feature of severe ulcerative colitis.

4.68 Investigations of the GI tract

1. D Colonoscopy

2. D Colonoscopy

In the first case scenario, one would suspect or need to exclude a colonic tumour, polyp or angiodysplasia. Thus, a colonoscopy would be the most appropriate investigation. In fact some people would advocate an initial colonoscopy anyway as this patient is in the at-risk age group for having colonic polyps/tumour.

The second clinical scenario represents a patient with a sigmoid volvulus, and the most appropriate investigation here would be a colonoscopy to decompress the volvulus. It is possible to perform a rigid sigmoidoscopy in the A&E department to achieve the same effect.

4.69 BDE

Perianal abscesses often start as an infection of the anal glands in the intersphincteric space. If these glands become infected and the ducts blocked, pus accumulates and may track in various directions producing a fistula. Anal fistulas, not abscesses, usually obey Goodsall's rule.

4.70 BCD

Obturator hernia occurs through the obturator canal. It is likely to strangulate because of the firm fibrous and bony edges around the neck. It is commoner in women >50 years who are thin and multiparous. It may present with small bowel obstruction. Patients usually hold the affected hip joint in semiflexion. A Prolene mesh placed in the preperitoneal space and sutured to Cooper's ligament is used for repair.

4.71 CDE

Other relations include the left kidney and adrenal (not the right), the body and tail of the pancreas (not the head). The transverse mesocolon and the spleen are also relations.

4.72 ADE

Relations include the right and left bronchi, the trachea, the vagus nerve, pleura, the aortic arch and descending aorta and the thoracic duct.

4.73 CEF

Scarpa's fascia is divided in a Kocher's incision. T10 corresponds to the umbilical area. The rectus sheath is deficient posteriorly only below the arcuate line, but is present in two layers in the subcostal region.

4.74 ACE

The lienorenal ligament connects the hilum of the spleen to the left kidney. It contains both the splenic artery and vein as well as the tail of the pancreas. The left adrenal gland lies slightly above and behind the ligament.

4.75 ABD

The incidence of diverticular disease increases with age. However, only 10% will become symptomatic. 90% of diverticula are located in the sigmoid colon and this is the exclusive site in 50%. When treated medically, diverticulitis recurs in 25% with the majority of recurrences occurring in the first 5 years. CT scan with contrast is sensitive and specific in looking for localised wall thickening >5 mm, inflammation of pericolic fat and abscess formation. Gastrografin enema will show segmental lumen narrowing and tethered mucosa. Both investigations will show extraluminal air/Gastrografin. A Hartmann's procedure is the safest option for perforation and faecal peritonitis. Colectomy and primary anastomosis has an 8% mortality, a 30% clinical leak rate and is not recommended in the presence of faecal peritonitis; however, some surgeons would perform such a procedure for purulent peritonitis.

4.76 CE

Anal cancer is uncommon, accounting for 4% of all large bowel malignancies. A history of genital warts (human papillomaviruses 6 and 11) increases the risk 25-fold. Although human papillomaviruses 16, 18, 31 and 33 are commonly associated with genital condylomas, they are more commonly found in high-grade intraepithelial neoplasia and invasive carcinomas. Anal cancer spreads locally in a cephalad direction. Lymph nodes occur frequently but only 50% have tumour deposits. Pain and bleeding are the most common presenting symptoms.

4.77 ABCE

Pancreatic pseudocysts are collections of fluid in the lesser sac, and they lack an epithelial lining. They occur in over 10% cases of pancreatitis as a result of duct disruption with leakage of pancreatic juice into the surrounding tissue. There is no natural border to the passage of pancreatic juice, therefore pseudocysts may occur anywhere from the mediastinum to the scrotum. Trauma may cause duct disruption leading to pseudocyst formation. The most reliable means of making a diagnosis is by ultrasound or CT scanning.

4.78 BCF

Described in 1955 – severe peptic ulcer disease, hypersecretion of gastric acid and non-β-islet-cell tumour of the pancreas. It occurs at all ages. 60% of gastrinomas are malignant. Most patients have ulcers in the duodenal bulb; however, multiple ulcers or in unusual locations should make one suspicious of Zollinger–Ellison syndrome, especially if associated with diarrhoea. CT and angiography are the mainstay investigations. Control of gastric acid can be controlled by H_2-antagonists and proton-pump inhibitors. Operative treatment includes curative resection of the gastrinoma and palliative reduction of tumour burden and gastrectomy.

4.79 BD

Most gallbladder cancers are incidental findings at histological examination of the gallbladder or with right hypochondrial pain. The 5-year survival rate is 5% and the only effective treatment is surgery. It is exceptionally rare in the absence of gallstones. Surgery is the only effective treatment.

4.80 ABC

Dumping syndrome may follow any form of gastric surgery. Early dumping syndrome presents with symptoms of epigastric discomfort, sweating and diarrhoea related to eating. This occurs due to passage of hyperosmolar solutions into the small bowel with fluid and potassium sequestration in the small intestine. Late dumping after 1–2 hours results from high plasma-insulin levels. This can be avoided by frequent meals low in carbohydrates and by pylorus-saving surgery.

4.81 Pancreatitis

1. B Acute-on-chronic pancreatitis
2. E Pancreatic pseudocyst
3. D Acute pancreatitis

The 43-year-old alcoholic with pain radiating to his back relieved by leaning forward is most likely to have chronic pancreatitis. A very similar picture can be seen with carcinoma of the head of the pancreas, but the one discriminating feature is that pain is constant and persistent in carcinoma. Moreover, the peak incidence of pancreatic adenocarcinoma is 60–80 years of age.

A patient who is alcoholic with a history of chronic pancreatitis and a palpable abdominal mass suggests a pancreatic pseudocyst. This can be easily diagnosed by ultrasound or CT scanning.

This final clinical case scenario is typical of acute pancreatitis with a history of sudden onset of pain, vomiting and an increased serum amylase level.

4.82 C

On digital per rectum examination, the structures that can be palpated in either sex are: the coccyx and lower sacrum behind; the ischial spines and ischiorectal fossae at the sides; and the anorectal ring at the anorectal junction. In the male, the prostate can be felt (but normal seminal vesicles are not usually palpable). In the female, the cervix can be felt through the vaginal wall, with the uterosacral ligaments laterally and sometimes the ovaries.

4.83 AE

The epiploic foramen of Winslow lies behind the free edge of the lesser omentum. The posterior wall of the epiploic foramen is formed by the peritoneum of the posterior abdominal wall, which passes as a smooth layer from the hepatorenal pouch to the duodenum. Behind this peritoneum lies the inferior vena cava. The superior border of the epiploic foramen is formed by the inferior surface of the liver (caudate lobe). The first part of the duodenum forms part of the inferior border. The portal vein lies anteriorly in the free edge of the opening.

4.84 All true

All these conditions may be cause of RUQ pain. Acute cholecystitis and gastritis can both cause epigastric and right upper quadrant pain in a woman of this age. Lobar pneumonia should also be suspected as a possible cause of right upper quadrant pain; a chest examination together with a CXR would exclude this. Ruptured ovarian cysts may cause RUQ pain. Chlamydia or gonococcal infection may cause a perihepatitis (Fitz-Hugh–Curtis syndrome) and therefore RUQ discomfort.

4.85 ABC

Splenectomy is associated with increased susceptibility to capsulate organisms including *Pneumococcus* and *Meningococcus* spp. and *Haemophilus influenzae.* Thrombocytosis (platelet count >600 x 10^9/l) may occur after splenectomy, peaking after 7 days. Although the short gastric arteries (arising from the splenic artery) are at risk, the stomach has an excellent blood supply from other vessels – the right and left gastroepiploic arteries and right and left gastric arteries.

4.86 CDF

The irritable bowel syndrome is a functional bowel disorder producing symptoms of abdominal pain, bloating, altered bowel habit (diarrhoea, constipation, or a mixture of both diarrhoea and constipation) and faecal urgency. It does not cause large bowel obstruction. Solitary rectal ulcer is a condition that is seen in patients with rectal evacuatory difficulty/dissatisfaction. Ulcerative colitis is an inflammatory condition affecting the mucosa of the large bowel and does not cause mechanical obstruction. However, Crohn's disease is a well-recognised cause of colonic strictures and hence obstruction. Diverticular disease can lead to stricture formation and hence large bowel obstruction, but is relatively uncommon.

4.87 Cholecystectomy

1. D ERCP

2. B Elective cholecystectomy

An ERCP is a useful method of removing stones from the common bile duct to relieve jaundice. It is associated with a 1% risk of pancreatitis and a 0.1% risk of mortality.

If patients are fit enough and are symptomatic from gallstones, then a cholecystectomy should be performed. Nearly 90% of all cholecystectomies are performed laparoscopically in the UK.

4.88 Pancreatic tumour
1. C Insulinoma
2. A Zollinger–Ellison syndrome

Insulinomas produce episodes of hypoglycaemia leading to altered behaviour and disturbances of consciousness. Characteristically, the patient feels well between episodes. It is a difficult diagnosis to make unless there is a degree of clinical suspicion.

In the second case, the patient has MEN-1. The hypercalcaemia arises from hyperparathyroidism. He also has Zollinger–Ellison syndrome as part of this syndrome, which causes markedly raised levels of gastrin and gastric acid hypersecretion. This gives rise to severe ulceration not only in the stomach and duodenum but also the jejunum.

4.89 ACE

The first stem should not be confused with the suspensory ligaments of the breast also known as the ligaments of Cooper. The duct of Santorini is the accessory pancreatic duct. The transversalis fascia and Scarpa's fascia are not related structures. Cloquet's node lies in the medial compartment of the femoral sheath where a small anatomical empty space exists and femoral hernias can occur. Alcock's canal is a fascial tunnel on the lateral wall of the ischiorectal fossa which conveys the pudendal nerve and vessels.

4.90 ABC

The bare area of the liver is in direct contact with the right suprarenal gland and the diaphragm. The right suprarenal gland extends medially behind the IVC, separated from the 12th rib by the diaphragm. It typically has three arterial sources. It receives blood from the inferior phrenic, from a branch of the renal artery and from a branch directly from the aorta. The venous drainage is into the inferior vena cava by a very short vessel. The left suprarenal gland drains into its corresponding renal vein.

4.91 AB

The pancreas is an essential endocrine organ that produces insulin, glucagon and other hormones. Pancreatic secretion is alkaline and is to maintain the correct pH levels for enzyme action and function. The exocrine function of the pancreas is to produce enzymes for normal digestion. Inactive precursors of these enzymes are secreted in pancreatic juice and cleaved to form trypsin, chymotrypsin, as well as carboxypeptidases, lipase, co-lipase and amylase. Secretion of pancreatic juice is primarily under the control of two hormones – secretin and cholecystokinin (CCK) secreted by the duodenum. The rate of pancreatic secretion is typically 150 ml/h and therefore approximately 3500 ml/day.

4.92 CD

Ulcerative colitis does not usually necessitate a total colectomy at a young age. Only in complicated cases (i.e. when there is an acute exacerbation with toxic dilatation, perforation, haemorrhage, failure to thrive, or malignant change) should total colectomy be necessary. This need for total colectomy below the age of 25 years is extremely rare. Steroids are used to control an acute exacerbation but not for maintenance of remission. For maintenance of remission, 5-aminosalicylic acid derivatives are used (sulfasalazine, mesalazine, olsalazine and balsalazide). Panproctocolitis involves the whole of the large bowel, and may give rise to a 'backwash' ileitis.

4.93 BE

Other differentials include lymph node, femoral artery aneurysm and lipoma. A spigelian hernia appears in the abdominal wall at the level of the arcuate line near the iliac crest through the site of weakness where the internal oblique contributes to the anterior and posterior sheath. A psoas abscess is usually tubercular in origin and presents in the femoral triangle. Troisier's node is an enlarged left supraclavicular lymph node, originally described to represent a metastasis from a gastric cancer. However, a Troisier's node may occur in other intra-abdominal malignancies such as pancreatic and colonic carcinomas. It is also seen in breast and lung cancers.

4.94 CE

Neural and hormonal signals control pancreatic exocrine secretion. The main trigger is the presence of acid and products of digestion in the duodenum, not the presence of triglycerides. Lipase is secreted by glands near the base of the tongue (responsible for up to 30% of triglyceride digestion), and the remainder is digested by pancreatic lipase – which requires a cofactor (co-lipase) to become active. The products of triglyceride breakdown are free fatty acids and 2-monoglycerides

4.95 Side-effects of treatment for inflammatory bowel disease

1. E Metronidazole
2. A Sulfasalazine
3. B Corticosteroids
4. B Corticosteroids
5. C Methotrexate
6. C Methotrexate

As well as nausea and vomiting, metronidazole may cause peripheral neuropathy, convulsions, headaches and hepatitis. Metronidazole is associated with irreversible peripheral neuropathy and does not appear to be related to the dose or length of time of ingestion.

The hepatic fibrosis and pneumonitis from methotrexate use is related to the total dose given. Other adverse effects include myelosuppression, nausea and vomiting, stomatitis, diarrhoea, osteoporosis, renal dysfunction, acute vasculitis (if high doses used) and seizures (especially after intrathecal use).

Osteoporosis and cataracts are well-known complications of corticosteroids. Other effects include susceptibility to infection, cushingoid appearance, central obesity, buffalo hump, moon facies, diabetes, hypertension, peptic ulceration, thin and easily bruised skin, striae, mental changes and proximal myopathy.

4.96 Surgical investigations

1. A Gastrografin enema
2. E Abdominal ultrasound
3. B Abdominal and pelvic CT scan
4. C small bowel follow-through
5. A Gastrografin enema

An acutely obstructing large bowel cancer is best assessed with a gastrografin (water soluble) enema. This is because use of barium in the enema may result in a severe peritonitis if it leaks through a bowel perforation into the peritoneum. Colonoscopy is associated with an increased risk of perforation.

A barium enema clearly defines the presence and extent of colonic diverticular disease, but a CT scan would identify an abscess associated with diverticular disease.

Mesenteric fat stranding and localised inflammatory changes would be seen with a CT scan. Acute and chronic gallbladder pathology is best seen on ultrasound.

Small bowel pathology is presently not well imaged by other forms of investigation other than follow-through contrast examinations.

Early colonic anastomotic leaks are best assessed using Gastrografin enemas or CT.

4.97 Surgical investigations
1. B Abdominal CT scan
2. C Small bowel follow-through
3. F Barium enema (double contrast)
4. B Abdominal CT scan

No technique is certain to reveal a colovesical fistula, but cystoscopy and barium enema are the two most likely investigations to help (one may see air in the bladder). X-ray of spun urine following a barium enema may also reveal barium radio-opacity. Pancreatic necrosis is not well visualised on ultrasound. Dynamic CT scans will usually demonstrate non-perfused pancreatic tissue.

4.98 Abdominal disease
1. D Familial adenomatous polyposis
2. C Ulcerative colitis
3. A Crohn's disease
4. A Crohn's disease
5. C Ulcerative colitis
6. B Diverticular disease

Desmoid tumours are benign proliferations of well-differentiated fibroblasts. They classically occur in the lower rectus sheath and infiltrate the surrounding tissues. They are associated with intestinal tumours and Gardner's syndrome (multiple osteomas and familial adenomatous polyposis).

Enteroenteric fistulas are more likely to complicate Crohn's disease than diverticular disease. Diverticular disease accounts for approximately half of all colovesical fistulas, and Crohn's disease comprises only about 15–20%. Pyoderma gangrenosum, ankylosing spondylitis and toxic megacolon are more common in ulcerative colitis than in Crohn's disease. Anal pathology is much more prevalent in Crohn's disease.

4.99 Hernias
1. D Lumbar hernia
2. E Gluteal hernia
3. G Perineal hernia
4. B Spigelian hernia

Lumbar hernias occur through either the inferior lumbar triangle of Petit (bounded by the iliac crest, the posterior edge of the external oblique and the anterior edge of the latissimus dorsi) or the superior lumbar space (bounded by the 12th rib, the lower border of the serratus posterior inferior as well as the anterior border of the sacrospinalis and the internal oblique). A perineal hernia is seen as a rare complication of A-P resection, and develops through a non-healing perineal wound.

4.100 AD

The neck of a femoral hernia is narrower and less accommodating than that of the internal inguinal ring, hence it more frequently presents with strangulation. Femoral hernias are more commonly found in women than men, but as a whole inguinal hernias are more common than femoral in women. Up to 85% of inguinal hernias are suitable for repair as a day-case procedure. The most commonly performed technique for inguinal hernia repair in adults is the Lichtenstein mesh technique. The Shouldice repair is an acceptable alternative. Children (<12 years old) are usually treated by herniotomy and suture repair. Large incarcerated inguinoscrotal hernias in older patients may require sacrifice of the cord structures, with subsequent orchidectomy.

4.101 BCD

Inguinal hernia may be repaired under local or general anaesthesia. A herniotomy would not be appropriate in a man but would be suitable for repair of an inguinal hernia in children under 12 years old. Laparoscopic extraperitoneal repair is an acceptable treatment in experienced hands (though it is not approved by NICE), but the long-term results are unknown. The Bassini repair (or nylon darn) has fallen out of favour, due to higher rates of recurrence compared to the Shouldice or tension-free mesh repairs.

4.102 ACD

Scarpa's fascia is incised during the surgical approach to an inguinal hernia. The iliohypogastric nerve supplies the internal oblique and transversus, and may be divided during an appendicectomy which may lead to a direct inguinal hernia. The iliohypogastric nerve is not encountered during normal inguinal hernia repair. However, the ilioinguinal nerve is usually seen. The nerve supplies cutaneous sensation to the skin at the base of the penis and part of the scrotum. Scarpa's fascia where it continues over the penis and scrotum assumes a different name: superficial perineal fascia of Colles. The superior epigastric vein drains the rectus muscle and enters the internal thoracic veins.

4.103 ACD

Following a meal, cholecystokinin is secreted by the duodenum and stimulates contraction of the gallbladder and relaxation of the sphincter of Oddi, thus allowing bile to enter the duodenum. Bile salts are involved in the absorption of fat through the formation of micelles. Bile salts are absorbed in the terminal ileum and transported back to the liver. This forms part of the enterohepatic circulation and prevents excessive loss of bile salts. Bile salts have a stimulating action on the gut, increasing mobility and thereby decreasing bowel transit times. Failure to absorb bile salts will cause diarrhoea.

4.104 ABCDFG

Chronic alcohol abuse may cause a Wernicke's encephalopathy (a reversible condition) and Korsakoff's syndrome (irreversible). Signs and symptoms of cerebellar ataxia are common in chronic alcoholism. Other effects of chronic alcohol ingestion include generalised marrow depression, with lymphopenia and immunosuppression. Macrocytosis is generally due to decreased folate level caused by chronic alcohol abuse. Sydenham's chorea is associated with rheumatic fever.

4.105 ABCE

Crohn's disease is a granulomatous inflammatory disorder involving the whole thickness of the bowel wall (any part of the GI tract from mouth to anus). Ulcerative colitis (UC) is a non-granuloma process that only involves the mucosa. This difference may explain the higher incidence of stricture, obstruction and fistula formation in Crohn's disease. UC invariably involves the rectum and extends proximally towards the caecum, and can sometimes cause a 'backwash ileitis'. Perianal problems (fissures, fistulas, skin tags) are much more commonly seen in Crohn's disease than UC.

4.106 CDE

The terminal ileum is the most common site of GI involvement in Crohn's disease (affects 60–70% of cases). Crohn's disease is characterised by skip lesions, cobblestone mucosa and rose-thorn ulceration. Extraintestinal manifestations include erythema nodosum, clubbing, pyoderma gangrenosum arthropathy and uveitis. Erythema multiforme is an ulcerative immunological condition occurring in response to a drug allergy.

4.107 ACDE

A rectus sheath haematoma may occur when there is sudden forceful contraction of the rectus muscle producing a tear of the superior or inferior epigastric vessels. This may occur as a result of direct injury, e.g. following a seat-belt injury, prolonged fits of coughing or sneezing, or physical exertion (e.g. in athletes). However, it may also occur spontaneously, and has a higher incidence in people on anticoagulant therapy. Rectus sheath haematoma is usually diagnosed on ultrasound scanning. Haematoma of the rectus sheath is usually treated conservatively with rest and analgesia.

However, if there is progressive pain and swelling, surgical evacuation is warranted and the bleeding point ligated. The presentation of a rectus sheath haematoma may mimic intra-abdominal pathology. Therefore, a careful history and examination with radiological investigation are needed to establish the correct diagnosis.

4.108 Polyps

1. E Inflammatory polyps
2. C Peutz–Jeghers' polyps
3. B Villous adenomatous polyps
4. B Villous adenomatous polyps
5. A Tubular adenomatous polyps

Villous adenomas of the rectum frequently present with the passage of bright-red blood and mucus per rectum. If villous adenomas are large, mucus secretion is significant and hypokalaemia may occur. Villous adenomas have the greatest malignant potential of all colorectal polyps. Peutz–Jeghers' polyps have no malignant potential themselves, but are associated with an increased risk of other malignant gut polyps.

Metaplastic polyps are also known as hyperplastic polyps. They are symptomless, occurring throughout the large bowel and are the most common type of polyp found in the rectum. They are thought not to undergo dysplastic or neoplastic change. Inflammatory polyps have no malignant potential.

4.109 Gastrointestinal haemorrhage

1. B Oesophagogastroduodenoscopy
2. A Colonoscopy
3. A Colonoscopy

Any patient who attends the A&E department with a massive fresh bleed per rectum that causes haemodynamic compromise should undergo an oesophagogastroduodenoscopy to exclude a bleeding peptic ulcer. Only after this has been excluded should one proceed with lower GI investigations.

In the second case, the elderly man is not in shock and the nature of the bleeding is suggestive of a lower GI cause – e.g. diverticular disease or colonic carcinoma. In this instance a colonoscopy would probably be the best first-line investigation.

In the third case, the young man who presents to the clinic with no local cause for his rectal bleeding should undergo a colonoscopy to exclude a polyp. This investigation is preferable to a barium enema as it may be therapeutic as well as diagnostic and has a higher specificity and sensitivity. The use of CT colonography for the screening of polyps and colonic cancer is presently undergoing evaluation.

4.110 Hernias

1. E **Pantaloon hernia**
2. C **Maydl's hernia**
3. D **Sliding hernia**
4. A **Richter's hernia**
5. B **Littre's hernia**

In a sliding hernia the posterior wall of the hernial sac is formed by a herniating viscus. This is usually sigmoid colon or bladder. Particular care is required during repair not to injure the herniated viscus, which can be seen when examining inside the opened sac.

4.111 ACDEF

Faecal impaction produces overflow incontinence. The mechanisms are unclear but may involve reflex relaxation of the internal sphincter leading to passive faecal soiling. Postpartum obstetric injuries are a major cause of faecal incontinence and may occur in up to 30% of births. This is dependent on the size of the baby, whether the delivery was assisted (e.g. forceps delivery) and if any tears occurred. It is important to note that faecal incontinence may present soon after the birth of the baby, but in many instances may occur years later. Pelvic radiotherapy may lead to decreased compliance and fibrosis of the rectum and postirradiation proctitis, all mechanisms that can cause faecal incontinence.

4.112 Jaundice

1. A **Duodenal carcinoma**
2. D **Acute cholangitis**
3. B **Biliary colic**

Patient 1 has FAP. Such patients have adenomas in the colon and duodenum. The commonest extraintestinal manifestation of FAP is a duodenal carcinoma. The presence of a duodenal carcinoma should be suspected in a patient with FAP who becomes jaundiced. The tumour here appears to be causing extrahepatic biliary obstruction.

Patient 2 exhibits altered features of Charcot's triad: fever, pain and rigors. Cholangitis is usually the result of a stone in the common bile duct.

Patient 3 is most likely to have biliary colic, as this does not usually cause jaundice.

4.113 AC

The incidence of abdominal wound dehiscence varies from 0.2 to 3% of abdominal wounds, and is more frequent after emergency surgery. Dehiscence affects male patients more often than females (4–5:1). Midline incisions are more likely to disrupt than transverse, but controlled trials of elective surgery have shown no difference in the dehiscence rate from paramedian incisions. The choice of suture material is critical: non-absorbable material (e.g. nylon) or absorbable material with prolonged tensile strength (PDS) should be used. Closure of the peritoneal layer is not critical.

4.114 BDE

The incidence of oesophageal cancer has been rising more rapidly over the past two decades. Presentation is usually at an advanced stage and hence the overall 5-year survival rate is 10%. The survival rate may rise to 50% for early-stage node-negative disease. Barrett's oesophagus may be complicated by adenocarcinoma. The risk of this complication depends upon the degree of cytological dysplasia.

Neoadjuvant and adjuvant radiotherapy and chemotherapy have had a limited effect on prognosis.

4.115 BCD

Sigmoid volvulus occurs following an anticlockwise torsion. A plain abdominal X-ray will confirm the diagnosis in 80% cases. Features on X-ray include: coffee-bean signs, beak sign at the site of torsion and an elevated diaphragm. Sigmoid colectomy with primary anastomosis or a Hartmann's procedure are indicated for cases with gangrene or perforation. It is controversial whether one procedure is superior to the other, but one-stage sigmoid colectomy is currently favoured.

4.116 A

Gardner's syndrome is a variant of familial adenomatous polyposis which is inherited in an autosomal dominant fashion. HPV is associated with anal and cervical cancer. Colonic lesions arising in the right colon tend to present at a later stage than lesions in the left colon. Left colonic tumours usually present with rectal bleeding or obstruction. Right colonic lesions often present with microcytic anaemia and/or an abdominal mass. Radiotherapy and chemotherapy (5-FU) are recognised treatment modalities for colonic carcinoma.

4.117 Jaundice
1. E Empyema of the gallbladder
2. C Common bile-duct stone
3. D Mucocele of the gallbladder

A palpable right upper quadrant mass, fever and the feeling of being generally unwell would point to an empyema of the gallbladder.

Obstructive jaundice 48 hours after open cholecystectomy is most likely to be due to common bile duct (CBD) calculus, which was missed at the time of surgery. This could have been avoided if a preoperative ultrasound had shown dilatation of the CBD from stones, in which case the stones would have been visualised and removed by preoperative ERCP.

Alternatively, during an open cholecystectomy, an intraoperative cholangiogram can be performed to visualise stones in the CBD. The CBD can then be opened, the stones removed and a T-tube left *in situ.*

A stone in Hartmann's pouch causing right quadrant upper pain is most likely to lead to a mucocele.

4.118 ABE

Rectal carcinoma, especially if low- or mid-rectal, may be treated with a course of preoperative radiotherapy to reduce local recurrence and reduce the tumour volume, thereby making an inoperable tumour resectable. The correct selection criteria and precise guidelines are as yet unknown. Rectal carcinoma, like colonic carcinoma, is thought to originate from polyps and only when they enlarge do they ulcerate. Rectal cancer spreads via lymphatics along the blood vessels (inferior mesenteric) to the para-aortic nodes. 5-Fluorouracil has been used in conjunction with other agents including folinic acid for Dukes C carcinoma. It is presently unclear whether chemotherapy should be given to patients with Dukes B rectal cancers. However, chemotherapy is not indicated for Dukes A carcinoma.

4.119 CDE

Diazepam is a long-acting benzodiazepine with a half-life exceeding 24 hours; it is broken down into active metabolites, hence its long half-life. Its effects are reversed by flumazenil. Naloxone reverses the effects of opiates. Antegrade amnesia is produced by diazepam.

4.120 Pancreatic tumours
1. B Glucagonoma
2. C Insulinoma

Glucagonomas are rare, but present with long-standing eczematous rash (usually >1 year), glossitis, stomatitis, diabetes and wasting.
Clinical features of insulinoma include disturbances of consciousness and 'odd' behaviour; in fact almost any neurological or psychiatric syndrome can be mimicked. Conversation and movement may be restricted during attacks, but the patient feels normal between attacks. It is part of the MEN-1 syndrome.
Both glucagonomas and insulinomas should be treated surgically becuase of the malignant potential of these tumours.

4.121 AE

The gastrointestinal tract is selectively impaired in patients who are in shock. It is one of the first organs to be affected and one of the last to be restored by resuscitation. Measurement of stomach perfusion can be estimated on the basis of the intramural pH. It is measured by tonometry: a catheter is filled with saline and allowed to equilibrate with the luminal PCO_2, which is assumed to be the same as the PCO_2 of the superficial mucosa. Determination of the arterial bicarbonate concentration will allow calculation of the intramural pH using the Henderson–Hasselbalch equation. This measurement reflects splanchnic tissue oxygenation and is an indirect and early means of estimating global tissue oxygenation.

4.122 BE

The caudate lobe (segment I according to Couinaud's 1957 classification) lies posterior to the portal vein but anterior to the inferior vena cava. Three main hepatic veins divide the liver into four sectors each of which receives a portal pedicle, with an alternation between hepatic veins and portal pedicles. According to this functional anatomy, the liver is divided into hemi-livers (right and left) by the main portal scissura called Cantlie's line.

4.123 E

Selection of patients for a pouch is important as complications occur in 30–50% of cases. Contraindications, at present, include those with Crohn's disease, particularly if there is any pelvic sepsis. Most surgeons routinely defunction to mitigate the effects of any pelvic sepsis, but this is usually with a loop ileostomy. A radiographic contrast study, 'pouchogram' is usually performed after 8 or more weeks to assess for any leaks prior to ileostomy reversal. Pelvic sepsis occurs in approximately 30% of cases and is the most common complication of this procedure. Frequency of defecation following a 'successful' ileoanal pouch is usually between 4 and 8 episodes/day.

4.124 D

An anal fissure is a linear ulcer which occurs in the anal canal just distal to the dentate line and classically causes pain on defecation with bleeding. The treatment of anal fissure involves conservative measures including dietary manipulation and stool softeners. Chemical sphincterotomy may be achieved by the use of topical nitrates, and more recently calcium antagonists such as diltiazem have been used. Botulinum toxin has also been shown to be successful (reported rates of 70%). If surgery is required then a lateral sphincterotomy may be performed. This is usually limited to the extent of the fissure. However, in a lateral sphincterotomy there is the risk of passive faecal incontinence as the internal sphincter is divided. An advancement flat is often regarded as a superior alternative. Some 80% of fissures usually occur in the posterior position in men and 60% in women. Anal fissure is associated with Crohn's disease more than ulcerative colitis. Anal fissure is not a premalignant condition, as opposed to anal condylomas which are related to anal carcinoma.

4.125 Jaundice

1. C Posthepatic jaundice
2. B Hepatic jaundice
3. C Posthepatic jaundice
4. C Posthepatic jaundice

Associations with prehepatic jaundice include the presence of urinary urobilinogen and the absence of urinary bilirubin. Causes include recent blood transfusion and a family history of haemolytic syndromes.

Hepatic jaundice may be conjugated or unconjugated. Causes include a history of recent foreign travel, alcohol or drug abuse, ingestion of hepatotoxic drugs (halothane, chlorpromazine) or liver tumours.

Associations with posthepatic jaundice include bilirubin in the urine, a positive Courvoisier's sign (extrahepatic duct obstruction), pruritus, a history of fever, jaundice and rigors (Charcot's triad – due to cholangitis) and a history of dark urine and pale stools.

4.126 ACDE

The levator ani forms part of the deep external anal sphincter. The anal canal has no longitudinal muscular coat. Lymph from the lower anal canal drains via the superficial inguinal nodes. The entire anal sphincter is innervated by the inferior rectal branch of the pudendal nerve (S2–S4). The upper anal canal is thrown into vertical folds called anal columns. The anal valves are formed by horizontal semilunar folds of mucous membrane joining adjacent columns at their lower end. Anal valves are remnants of the proctodeal membrane. The anococcygeal body lies between the anal canal and the coccyx.

4.127 CD

The veins in the mesentery are all tributaries of the portal system. The root of the small bowel mesentery extends from a point to the left of the L2 vertebra, at the duodenojejunal junction, down to the right sacroiliac joint. The nerves are postganglionic sympathetic and preganglionic parasympathetic fibres (CN X) from the superior mesenteric plexus. The superior mesenteric artery supplies the mid-gut, which includes the large bowel as far as the distal transverse colon. The transverse mesocolon lies anterior to the small bowel mesentery.

4.128 Rectal bleeding

1. **A Crohn's disease**
2. **G Meckel's diverticulum**
3. **B Solitary juvenile polyp**
4. **C Familial adenomatous polyposis**
5. **H Mid-gut volvulus**

Rectal bleeding is a common symptom throughout childhood.

Crohn's disease may present in many ways but is frequently associated with weight loss or linear growth failure in children.

Meckel's diverticulum may present with acute GI haemorrhage leading to the typical brick-red coloured stool. The ulceration is caused by the ectopic gastric mucosa within the Meckel's diverticulum and may also cause lower abdominal pain.

Solitary juvenile polyps are a relatively common cause of painless rectal bleeding. Occasionally juvenile polyps may be multiple.

Familial adenomatous polyposis should be suspected in children presenting with rectal bleeding when there is a family history of early colorectal carcinoma in immediate family members. The polyps generally develop after puberty.

Mid-gut volvulus is frequently preceded by a history of intermittent colicky abdominal pain with or without bile-stained vomiting – usually from the age of 3 months. This diagnosis should always be considered in a child with bile-stained vomiting and rectal bleeding.

4.129 ADE

Severe acute pancreatitis may lead to multiorgan failure and DIC. When the disease process continues for longer than 10 days, the development of a pseudocyst becomes more likely. However, most cases of pancreatitis are uncomplicated. Pancreatitis may be associated with a fall in the serum calcium level, although it may remain normal. Congenital pancreatic abnormalities, such as pancreas divisum or an annular pancreas, increase the likelihood of developing pancreatitis, the symptoms of which include pain radiating through to the back which is relieved by sitting forward. The important differential diagnosis is a leaking abdominal aortic aneurysm.

4.130 Abdominal pain

1. A Renal adenocarcinoma
2. C Pelviureteric obstruction
3. D Leaking abdominal aortic aneurysm

The presentation of the first patient is classically that of renal carcinoma; however, this triad of symptoms and signs only occurs in 30% of cases.
The loin pain in the patient who drinks four cups of coffee before work is most likely to be due to pelvic-ureteric obstruction. Symptoms of ureteric obstruction in adults usually occur after a fluid overload.
Any male patient above the age of 55 years who presents with back pain should be suspected of having a leaking abdominal aortic aneurysm (AAA) until proven otherwise, as AAAs are more common in this age group than urinary stones.

4.131 ABCE

The spleen lies on the diaphragm, separated from the 9th to 11th ribs by the costodiaphragmatic recess. The left extremity of the lesser sac extends into the hilum. The peritoneal fold called the lienorenal ligament (which contains the splenic vessels and the tail of the pancreas touching the spleen) passes from the left kidney to the spleen. Another peritoneal fold called the gastrosplenic ligament carries the short gastric and gastroepiploic vessels and joins the kidney to the stomach. The spleen is not palpable in the healthy individual, and must at least triple in size before it appears in the left hypochondrium.

4.132 ACD

The femoral sheath is a downward continuation of abdominal fascia about 2.5 cm below the inguinal ligament. It is believed to allow for femoral vessel movement in the inguinal region during movement of the hip. The mnemonic NAVEL describes some of the key structures in this region (from lateral to medial): femoral **n**erve, **a**rtery, **v**ein, **e**mpty space, **l**ymphatics (i.e. Cloquet's). Apart from the femoral nerve that lies most lateral, all the other structures in the mnemonic are encased in the femoral sheath. The mentioned empty space and lymphatic compartments form the 'femoral canal' where femoral hernias may occur. Therefore, the femoral canal is in the most medial portion of the femoral sheath. The femoral ring is the abdominal opening into the femoral canal. At 2–3 cm below the inguinal ligament, the femoral sheath fuses with the adventitia of the femoral vessels. The pubic branch of the inferior epigastric artery replaces the obturator artery in about 30% of cases, and may be at risk in a femoral hernia repair.

ANSWERS – CHAPTER 5: URINARY SYSTEM AND RENAL TRANSPLANTATION

5.1 ADF

In the male, the deep perineal pouch contains the membranous urethra, sphincter urethra, bulbourethral glands, deep transverse perineal muscles, internal pudendal vessels and dorsal nerves of the penis. The bulb of the penis lies in the superficial perineal pouch.

5.2 Loin pain

1. B Pyelonephritis
2. A Urinary calculi
3. B Pyelonephritis

One would suspect pyelonephritis in a male patient with loin pain, pyrexia and tachycardia.

In an 18-year-old man with right iliac fossa pain and microscopic haematuria one would suspect appendicitis or a urinary calculus. With a perforated appendicitis, however, the patient lies still, unlike the writhing around with the pain of ureteric colic.

The diagnosis would most likely be a pyelonephritis in view of the bilateral reflux, dysuria, malaise and fever in patient 3.

5.3 E

The lower edge of the external oblique aponeurosis is folded back on itself between the anterior superior iliac spine (ASIS) and pubic tubercle forming the inguinal ligament. The inguinal canal contains the ilioinguinal nerve (L1) and the genital branch of the genitofemoral nerve (L1–L2). The ilioinguinal nerve enters the inguinal canal via its anterior wall (not the deep ring) and runs outside the spermatic cord. The inferior epigastric artery marks the medial boundary of the deep inguinal ring. The deep inguinal ring is midway between the ASIS and pubic tubercle. Branches of the pudendal nerve (S2–S4) enter the perineum through the lesser sciatic foramen.

5.4 BCEG

The external (or superficial) inguinal ring is formed by a V-shaped defect in the external oblique aponeurosis above and medial to the pubic tubercle. It transmits the spermatic cord with all its contents plus the ilioinguinal nerve. The following are the contents of the spermatic cord: three fascial layers (external spermatic, cremasteric, internal spermatic); three arteries (testicular, cremasteric, vas deferens); pampiniform plexus, veins from the cremaster and vas deferens; and genital branch of the genitofemoral nerve, sympathetic fibres, vas deferens and lymphatics.

5.5 CDE

Horseshoe kidney is more common in men. The anatomical location and blood supply is very variable. They are more prone to infection and calculi formation due to relative upper tract stasis. They are also more prone to trauma.

5.6 Scrotal swellings

1. **C Varicocele**
2. **G Testicular tumour**
3. **F Inguinoscrotal hernia**
4. **A Hydrocele**

The classical history of a varicocele is the sensation of a bag of worms in the scrotum. The varicosities are more prominent when the patient is standing, and they disappear or decrease in size when the patient lies down.

An indirect inguinal hernia is more likely to occur on the right, as the right testis descends later. However, 98% of varicoceles occur on the left; reasons for this include: (1) the left testicular vein forms a greater angle with the left renal vein; (2) the left renal vein is crossed and may be compressed by the pelvic colon; (3) the left testicular vein is longer than the right; (4) the terminal valve is frequently absent in the left testicular vein.

The history of onset of testicular tumour is varied, but is often associated with the onset of sudden pain. One should always suspect a testicular tumour if an irregular testes is ever felt. An urgent ultrasound is required.

A painless, long-standing swelling that transilluminates within the scrotum is most likely to be a hydrocele. A hydrocele of the cord will be separate from the testis.

5.7 ABDE

Acute epididymitis is seen in all age groups but is rare before puberty. The infection reaches the epididymis via the bloodstream or retrograde from the prostatic urethra and seminal vesicles. Predisposing factors include UTI, STI and instrumentation of the urethra. Although *E. coli* is responsible for most infections, the causative organism varies with the age of the patient. In men <35 years *E. coli* is the responsible organism for most cases, whilst in children it is usually abacterial, being idiopathic or secondary to trauma. Late infection may be impossible to differentiate from torsion of the testis. In the long term, atrophy of the testis occurs in 20% of patients and fertility may be impaired.

5.8 BCD

Bladder calculi usually arise de novo in the bladder as a result of bladder outflow obstruction, diverticulae or foreign bodies. The classical picture is of sudden cessation of urinary stream during voiding with severe penile/perineal pain. Bladder calculi may be treated with extracorporeal shock wave lithotripsy (ESWL) but more commonly by endoscopic removal. Chronic urothelium irritation may lead to squamous metaplasia and squamous-cell carcinoma of the bladder.

5.9 ACE

Prostatic cancer has a rising incidence with age. Androgen suppression or androgen antagonists give symptomatic relief in disseminated carcinoma in about 75% of patients. Surgical castration reduces circulating androgen levels by about 95%.

5.10 Renal tract calculi

1. A Extracorporeal shock wave lithotripsy (ESWL)
2. C Nephrectomy
3. B Percutaneous nephrostomy

Stones measuring 2 cm in diameter, that lie within the kidney, are usually treated with ESWL. Percutaneous nephrolithotomy (PCNL) is used for a stone bulk >2 cm (or >1 cm in the lower pole calyx). ESWL can be used afterwards to residual fragments (called Steinstrasse, which have the appearance of a stone street in the ureter). Stones in the lower pole calyx have poor clearance rates and thus PCNL is the preferred option.

A staghorn calculus in a functional kidney is treated with PCNL followed by ESWL to remove residual fragments. However, in a patient with a 15% split function, the most appropriate treatment would be nephrectomy if the split function is <15%.

Obstructed infected kidneys need immediate drainage by percutaneous nephrostomy (from above).

Insertion of a ureteric stent (from below) is useful for preventing a stone causing a PUJ obstruction, for the prophylaxis of stones >1 cm prior to more definitive treatment and to keep luminal patency after accidental or planned ureteric opening.

5.11 BCD

The complications of TURP include hypothermia and transurethral syndrome. In the latter, absorption of the hypotonic irrigation solution leads to water intoxication and causes intravascular haemolysis, hyponatraemia and hypotension. Other complications include urethral stricture, incontinence (due to residual bladder instability), retrograde ejaculation and an increased risk of myocardial infarct 3 years post-TURP.

5.12 CD

Renal calculi usually present in early adult life, with two age peaks at 28 and 55 years. Common identifiable causes include idiopathic hypercalciuria (65%) and UTI (20%). Infective stones are staghorn calculi (Ca^{2+}, Mg^{2+}, NH_4PO_4) – formed by Enterobacteriaceae such as *Proteus* spp. which produce urease that splits urinary urea to form ammonium ions. Renal pelvic stones, if symptomatic and large, require ESWL, percutaneous nephrolithotomy or nephrectomy.

5.13 Benign prostatic hyperplasia
1. E Retropubic (open) prostatectomy
2. C TURP
3. C TURP

The morbidity in patients with very large prostates (>100 g) is less if open retropubic prostatectomy is performed rather than a TURP, as this reduces operation time and avoids excessive fluid absorption during prolonged surgery. Finasteride is a useful treatment in men with large (>40 g) prostates. It also reduces prostatic bleeding.

One must always warn a patient undergoing TURP of the risk of retrograde ejaculation following the operation.

Catheterisation is not indicated in simple chronic urinary retention unless renal function is impaired.

5.14 AB

Rupture of the spongy (penile) part of the urethra leaks urine into the superficial perineal fascia (of Colles), which is continuous with the membranous fascia (of Scarpa) in the anterior abdominal wall. The penile urethra takes a 90° angle through the bulbar part. The corpus spongiosum invests the penile urethra.

5.15 All true

The causes of neuropathic bladder dysfunction can be divided into cerebral lesions (e.g. CVA, dementia, parkinsonism), spinal lesions (e.g. trauma, multiple sclerosis, spina bifida) and peripheral nerve lesions (e.g. following pelvic surgery or diabetes mellitus). Lesions of the sacral cord or peripheral nerves cause an underactive detrusor and urethra. Lesions of the supraspinal cord cause loss of inhibitory impulses so causing detrusor overreactivity and uncoordinated activity of detrusor and urethra. Lesions above the pons cause loss of cerebral inhibition and may produce overactive detrusor. Detrusor and urethral activity remain uncoordinated.

5.16 Testicular tumours

1. D Radiotherapy

2. D Radiotherapy

3. G Retroperitoneal lymph node dissection

The present treatment of stage I seminoma is radical orchidectomy and prophylactic radiotherapy to the retroperitoneal nodes, although trials are under way comparing adjuvant radiotherapy with carboplatin (adjuvant chemotherapy). More advanced seminomas should be treated with chemotherapy also. Intratubular germ-cell neoplasia inevitably develops into cancer, therefore a prophylactic radiotherapy dose of 20 Gy is given to the remaining testis after sperm banking has been offered. The treatment of residual nodes following chemotherapy and normalisation of tumour markers is retroperitoneal lymph node dissection.

Teratomas are much less radiosensitive and should be treated by orchidectomy and platinum-based combination chemotherapy.

5.17 BC

Carcinoma of the prostate is the commonest adult male tumour in the USA where opportunistic screening is common. It is second to lung cancer in the UK. It is more common in African–Americans and in general in the black population. The risk is ninefold if two first-degree relatives are affected.

5.18 ACDE

Following TURP the causes of incontinence are usually a UTI or detrusor instability. Damage to the external sphincter is rare. TVT (transvaginal tape) is sited around the mid-urethra. A pelvic floor contraction may inhibit an involuntary detrusor contraction as well as strengthen the pelvic floor in those with stress incontinence.

5.19 Transitional-cell carcinoma

1. A TURBT

2. G Nephroureterectomy

3. D M-VAC chemotherapy

The diagnosis and treatment (in most cases) of a bladder tumour is a transurethral resection (TURBT) of the polypoid part of the tumour and biopsy to stage muscle invasion. If it is found to be stage T_2–T_{4a}, one should perform cystectomy ± radiotherapy, plus chemotherapy if preferred.

The standard treatment of a transitional-cell carcinoma in either the kidney or ureter is a nephroureterectomy, as these tumours are often multifocal and surveillance of a ureteric stump is difficult. A cystectomy is contraindicated if enlarged pelvic lymph nodes are detected preoperatively.

5.20 AC

Staghorn calculi (also known as struvite) are composed of magnesium, ammonium and phosphate. They form when urine pH >7. They are associated with *Proteus* spp. and other Gram-negative organisms which contain the enzyme urease. This results in the splitting of urea into ammonium ions, thus alkalinising the urine.

5.21 Imaging

1. **H Spiral CT scan**
2. **F DMSA scan**
3. **G DTPA scan**

A non-contrast spiral CT with thin cuts will detect 'all' calculi. This imaging modality may be used when an IVU or ultrasound are contraindicated or impractical. Staghorn calculi require DMSA imaging to ascertain the split function of the kidneys, as DMSA is secreted by the kidney. DTPA scans are used to show which kidney is obstructed, as it is filtered by the glomerulus. MAG-3 is filtered and secreted, and is now the most commonly used isotope in imaging departments.

PUJ obstruction has a trimodal distribution: antenatal, teenagers (when they start drinking alcohol) and the elderly. A diuresis in a patient with a PUJ obstruction worsens the pain and should arouse suspicion of this condition.

5.22 AD

PUJ obstruction is one of the more common disorders seen in infancy and childhood. It may occur as a result of intrinsic (morphological changes in smooth muscle and excess collagen), extrinsic or secondary causes (severe vesicoureteric reflux, urinary tract obstruction).

The male:female ratio is 5:2 and left:right is 5:2. PUJ obstruction is best detected with diuretic renography, i.e. DTPA or MAG-3 scanning with a diuretic, e.g. furosemide (frusemide). No intervention is necessary in utero unless there is oligohydramnios. Postnatally, a pyeloplasty should be carried out to preserve renal function if the abnormality persists.

5.23 ACE

The complete incontinence rate following radical prostatectomy is 2–5%. Cryotherapy is not a widely accepted treatment option for localised disease. Its use is mainly described in the treatment of salvage situations. Brachytherapy is the implantation of radioactive iodine or palladium seeds within the prostate.

5.24 Renal transplant
1. C Chronic rejection
2. A Acute rejection
3. D Blood group mismatch
4. B Hyperacute rejection

Hyperacute rejection occurs immediately, as result of a reaction from pre-existing antibodies to the transplanted tissue, e.g. ABO blood type mismatch.

Acute rejection occurs as a result of HLA type mismatch, and is controlled by matching donor and recipient HLA types and with immunosuppressive drugs.

The humoral immune system is responsible for chronic rejection, which can take months or years to occur.

5.25 DEF

Ejaculatory ducts enter the upper posterior part of the prostate gland to open into the urethra. Laterally lies the levator ani. The arterial supply to the prostate is derived from the inferior vesical artery, a branch entering the prostate at each side. The prostate is surrounded by a venous plexus, which drains into the internal iliac vein and subsequently into the internal vertebral venous plexus.

5.26 AD

The TNM classification is used to stage prostate cancer. T_1 is not palpable or visible. Tumours are stage T_{1a} if <5% chips are involved, and T_{1b} if >5% chips are involved following TURP. T2 is a tumour confined within the prostate. Extracapsular extension not involving the seminal vesicles is stage T_{3a}. Seminal vesicle involvement is stage T_{3b}. T_4 is when the tumour is fixed or invades adjacent structures.

PRACTICE PAPER 1 – MCQ ANSWERS

1 CD

Osteosarcoma is most commonly found at the metaphyses of long bones, and usually presents in the 2nd and 3rd decades of life. It is a rare but well-recognised complication of Paget's disease and this accounts for the second peak in incidence around the 6th decade. Osteosarcomas may be osteolytic, osteoblastic or show a mixed picture on X-ray. Sun-ray spicules represent new bone formation once the cortex has been destroyed. Bone formation in Codman's triangle is due to elevation of the periosteum by invasion of tumour through the cortex.

2 ACDE

The most common causes of conductive deafness include wax, acute otitis media, secretory otitis media, chronic otitis media, barotrauma, otosclerosis and injuries to the tympanic membrane and otitis externa. Less common causes include tumours of the middle ear and traumatic ossicular dislocation. Sensorineural deafness is caused by a number of causes including infections such as mumps, herpes zoster, meningitis and syphilis. Other causes of senorineural deafness include congenital–maternal rubella, cytomegalovirus, toxoplasmosis, prolonged exposure to loud noises, drugs (aspirin, aminoglycosides), Menière's disease, head injury and acoustic neuroma. Metabolic causes of sensorineural deafness include diabetes and hypothyroidism. In Paget's disease there may be a mixed hearing loss, i.e. conduction and sensorineural deafness. This may be due to ankylosis of the stapes, or compression on the VIIIth cranial nerve in the auditory foramen by bone.

3 CD

The posterior third of the tongue has no papillae but does contain the lingual (lymphoid) tonsil. The mucous membrane of the posterior third of the tongue is innervated by CN IX for both general and taste sensations. The very posterior of the dorsum of the tongue is innervated by the internal laryngeal nerve, a branch of the superior laryngeal nerve (CN X). The chordae tympani (CN VII) is the nerve for taste to the anterior two-thirds of the tongue.

4 ADEF

The ilioinguinal nerve (L1) emerges laterally to the psoas, descends posterior to the kidney and enters the inguinal canal by piercing the transversus abdominis and internal oblique muscles (not by passing through the deep ring). It then leaves the inguinal canal via the superficial inguinal ring. It is sensory to the skin of the lower abdomen and some of the genital area. The ilioinguinal (and iliohypogastric) nerves carry motor fibres to the external and internal obliques and the transversus abdominis. They travel in the anterior abdominal wall between the transversus and internal oblique muscles close to McBurney's point – so if they are damaged after a gridiron incision, they will paralyse the muscle fibres in the conjoint tendon and may give rise to an indirect inguinal hernia.

5 ABD

The colon absorbs up to 5 litres of water a day. The colonic mucosa actively absorbs sodium and chloride ions, whereas bicarbonate accumulates on the mucosal side. Chloride ions are actively absorbed against a large concentration gradient. Chloride and bicarbonate exchange has been estimated to provide 25% of total absorption in the colon. Short-chain fatty acids are produced by anaerobic fermentation of undigested carbohydrates by colonic bacteria.

6 DE

The rectum contains no mesentery by definition, although parts are covered by peritoneum. The pararectal lymph nodes drain into the inferior mesenteric and internal iliac nodes. The superior rectal vein drains into the inferior mesenteric vein (portal circulation). The middle rectal vein drains into the internal iliac vein and the inferior rectal vein drains into the internal pudendal vein (both systemic circulation). The arterial supply is principally from the superior rectal artery with contributions from the middle and inferior rectal and median sacral vessels.

7 AD

The causes of carpal tunnel syndrome include pregnancy, rheumatoid arthritis, hypothyroidism, osteoarthritis and fractures in the region of the wrist. The syndrome results from compression of the median nerve in the tunnel under the flexor retinaculum; if conservative measures fail, treatment is by surgical division of the flexor retinaculum. The nerve supplies motor fibres to the abductor pollicis brevis muscle. The differential diagnosis of carpal tunnel syndrome includes cervical rib and cervical spondylosis, which may produce similar symptoms.

8 CDG

Meckel's diverticulum occurs in 2% of the population and affects males twice as often as females. It is classically found 0.6 m from the ileocaecal valve on the antimesenteric border of the small intestine and is approximately 5 cm long. It is a true diverticulum with a mucous membrane and a muscular coat and may be connected to the umbilicus by either a fibrous band or a complete fistula – remnants of the vitellointestinal duct. Most cases of Meckel's diverticulum are asymptomatic, but 20% have heterotopic gastric or pancreatic mucosa. Complications of Meckel's diverticulum include diverticulitis, intussusception, ulceration and GI bleeding, intestinal obstruction and perforation. If a Meckel's diverticulum is found incidentally, it should be left alone, especially if it is non-inflamed with a wide neck.

9 ABCD

The kidneys lie retroperitoneally in the upper posterior abdominal wall. They are mostly covered by the costal margin. Both kidneys are in contact posteriorly with the costodiaphragmatic recess, psoas muscle, subcostal and ilioinguinal nerves. The cisterna chyli is found on the right of the aorta in front of L1 and L2. It is at a similar level to the kidneys and lies between them without direct contact.

10 AB

About 50% of enterovesical fistulas are secondary to diverticular disease, 15–20% are secondary to colorectal cancer, 15–20% are secondary to Crohn's disease and about 5% are secondary to bladder tumours. About 60% of patients have pneumaturia, and 30% have faecaluria.

11 CDE

Amyloidosis is a disorder where extracellular proteinaceous substances (protein fibrils) are deposited in body tissues, locally or systemically. Amyloidosis may be of primary or secondary aetiology, and is linked with chronic disease conditions that are usually inflammatory (rheumatoid arthritis, Crohn's disease) or caused by infections (TB); it is also associated with multiple myeloma, Hodgkin's disease and Waldenstrom's macroglobulinaemia. Other forms of amyloidosis are familial and isolated (e.g. Alzheimer's disease).

12 A

The femoral artery enters the thigh midpoint between the anterior superior iliac spine and the pubic symphysis. Here the femoral artery lies on the psoas major tendon which separates it from the capsule of the hip joint. The femoral artery emerges from the femoral canal and then courses downwards to disappear beneath the sartorius entering the adductor canal. Only the profunda femoris spirals deep to the adductor longus. At the adductor hiatus, the femoral vein is lateral but ascends posteriorly in the canal until it reaches the femoral triangle where it lies medial to the femoral artery. The femoral artery gives off a descending genicular artery whilst in the adductor canal.

13 ABE

The sural nerve branches off the tibial nerve in the popliteal fossa. It is usually joined by the sural communicating branch of the common peroneal nerve and supplies the back of the leg and the lateral foot. The tibial nerve enters the popliteal fossa lateral to the popliteal artery and then passes posterior then medial to the artery. Damage to the tibial nerve results in loss of plantar flexion of the feet.

14 BC

Males are more frequently complicated by acute glomerulonephritis following tonsillitis. This particular complication has a latency of 1–3 weeks.

Group A β-haemolytic streptococcal infection commonly occurs in children <10 years. Peritonsillar abscess or quinsy produce medial displacement of the soft palate and uvula. Pulmonary hypertension, CCF and secondary chronic hypoxia have all been described. Odynophagia and otalgia also occur.

Cholesteatoma is keratinised stratified squamous epithelium growing in the middle ear (which is usually lined by columnar epithelium). It should be treated aggressively as it can be invasive and fatal.

15 E

Pulmonary embolism produces a tachycardia and right ventricular heart strain, which may manifest as right bundle-branch block and right axis deviation. The classical ECG changes of $S_1Q_3T_3$ is rare. T-wave inversion in the right precordial leads may occur. Right atrial dilatation can cause prominent P waves in the inferior leads. Atrial fibrillation or flutter are common occurrences.

16 B

An epigastric hernia is a protrusion of abdominal contents between the interstices of the decussating fibres of the abdominal wall aponeuroses from the xiphoid process to the umbilicus. It is most common between the ages of 20 and 50 years. 20% are multiple but usually one is dominant. An epigastric hernia usually contains preperitoneal fat and is treated by direct surgical closure unless very large, when a mesh may be required.

17 ABEFG

The linea semilunaris marks the lateral margin of the rectus muscle and sheath passing from the pubic tubercle to the costal cartilage at the tip of the 9th rib, which overlies the fundus of the gallbladder on the right. The inferior epigastric vessels and medial umbilical ligament cross the linea posteriorly below the arcuate line before ascending in the posterior compartment of the rectus sheath. The anterior abdominal wall would be greatly weakened both physically and functionally by cutting along the semilunar line as the nerve supply to the rectus abdominis muscle and overlying skin would be interrupted. Furthermore, Langer's lines on the abdomen are horizontal. Spigelian hernias occur at the edge of the linea semilunaris, typically at the level of the arcuate line. The three borders of Hesselbach's triangle are the inferior epigastric artery, the inguinal ligament and the lateral border of the rectus abdominis muscle (linea semilunaris).

18 AE

Cystic fibrosis can cause intestinal obstruction due to the production of a very viscid meconium. It is an abnormality of the chloride ion channel, not calcium channels. 1:2000 live births are affected. Pancreatin (e.g. Creon) may be necessary in later in life to compensate for a reduced or absent exocrine pancreatic secretion.

19 E

Although the aromatic amines and other carcinogenic agents are a recognised cause of bladder cancer, the implementation of health and safety measures have made this a rarity. The commonest worldwide cause of bladder cancer is *Schistosoma haematobium*, but cigarette smoking is the leading causative agent in the West. TP53 mutations are associated with high-grade, muscle-invasive bladder cancers and with carcinoma in situ. The prognosis for carcinoma in situ is guarded, with approximately 50% developing muscle-invasive bladder cancer. Most bladder cancers (85%) are superficial and are treated endoscopically. Orthotopic bladder reconstruction causes metabolic abnormalities and therefore must not be used in patients with impaired renal function.

20 E

From superficial to deep, the scalp has five basic layers denoted by the mnemonic 'SCALP': **s**kin; **c**onnective tissue; **a**poneurosis; **l**oose areolar tissue; and **p**eriosteum. The blood supply to the scalp is from branches of both the internal and external carotid arteries. Two such tributaries from the internal carotid are the supraorbital and supratrochlear arteries. There is no C1 dermatome. The aponeurosis of the scalp is separated from the epicranium by loose connective tissue (the plane of cleavage in scalping) facilitating gliding movements. It contains no lymph nodes. Lymphatic drainage is mainly to the submandibular, preauricular, mastoid and occipital nodes. The occipitofrontalis muscle is supplied by CN VII.

21 AD

Extraintestinal manifestations of Gardner's syndrome include osteomas (especially of the skull and mandible), mesenteric and abdominal wall desmoids, lipomas, fibromas and epidermoid cysts. It is probably part of the same spectrum of disease to which FAP belongs, but it has more prominent extraintestinal manifestations.

22 ACE

The third part of the duodenum lies in the subcostal plane (L3) and follows the inferior margin of the pancreatic head. The third part of the duodenum lies posterior to the superior mesenteric vessels. It overlies the aorta and the beginning of the inferior mesenteric artery. The root of the small bowel mesentery is attached near its termination on the left. The second part of the duodenum overlies the right ureter and renal vessels in the hilum of the right kidney, separated from the renal artery by the vein.

23 ACE

Dupuytren's contracture is a thickening (with or without nodules) and contracture of the superficial palmar fascia. It is not related in any way to the flexor tendons themselves. Dupuytren's contracture is more common in men and in those with a history of alcoholism, diabetes or phenytoin therapy. Repetitive trauma is also an aetiological factor. Dupuytren's contracture tends to affect the ring and little fingers most frequently.

24 CDE

Maxillary carcinoma has a high mortality rate; 60% of cases present at an advanced stage. Pain, swelling and nasal obstruction are the more usual complaints. Proptosis develops if there is invasion of the orbit superiorly. Trismus occurs when the pterygoid palatal muscles become involved.

25 BD

The head of the pancreas is related to the hilum but does not overlie the right kidney. It is, however, anterior to the left kidney. The transpyloric plane (L1) transects the pancreas obliquely, passing through the midpoint of the neck, with most of the head below the plane, and most of the body and tail above. The transverse mesocolon is attached to the head, neck and body of the pancreas. The uncinate process lies posterior to the superior mesenteric vessels, and the inferior mesenteric vein passes behind the body of the pancreas, where it joins the splenic vein.

26 AC

The medial plantar nerve is a branch of the tibial nerve and supplies the medial three and a half toes on the plantar surfaces and the dorsal surfaces proximal to the nailbeds. The medial branch of the superficial peroneal nerve partly supplies the skin of the medial big toe and adjacent parts of the second and third toes.

27 CD

Postphlebitic syndrome results mainly from valvular destruction, post-thrombotic scarring and stiffening of the venous wall. Progression to this syndrome probably occurs as a result of popliteal- or more proximal-segment venous thrombosis. Complications of post-thrombotic syndrome/postphlebitic syndrome are very common in elderly people. Clinical features include swelling (usually due to accumulation of oedema fluid), subcutaneous fibrosis and induration as the disease progresses. Varicose eczema is also a feature, as is increased pigmentation due to deposition of haemosiderin in the tissues (lipodermatosclerosis).

28 BCDE

Metastatic prostate cancer is treated with hormonal therapy. Diethylstilbestrol is effective and is generally used as second-line treatment due to the risks of thrombosis (aspirin must be taken concomitantly).

Bicalutamide (Casodex) is a form of hormonal therapy for prostate cancer. It has a structure similar to testosterone and works by blocking and preventing the binding of testosterone to receptors on the surface of prostate cancer cells.

29 BDF

The nasopharynx lies behind the nasal cavity above the soft palate. The nasopharynx contains the pharyngeal tonsil (adenoid), salpingopharyngeal fold (produced by the salpingopharyngeus muscle), and the pharyngeal recess posterior to the tubal elevation and adjacent to the internal carotid artery. The pyramidal fossae lie in the laryngopharynx. The pharyngeal branch of the VII cranial nerve, coming from the pterygopalatine ganglion, supplies the mucosa of the nasopharynx.

30 BC

The most likely diagnosis is a thyroglossal cyst. Other diagnoses should include epidermal cyst and dermoid cyst. An ultrasound scan is the most useful first-line test. Treatment of thyroglossal cyst is by surgical excision.

31 ABD

The jejunum has a thicker wall, less mesenteric fat, more plicae circulares, a wider lumen, fewer Peyer's patches and fewer arterial arcades than the ileum.

32 BCD

Displaced intracapsular fractures of the femoral neck are usually treated with a hemiarthroplasty, although closed reduction and screw fixation may be appropriate in the young patient who has a good blood supply to the femoral head. An undisplaced fracture should be treated with screw fixation. Intertrochanteric (extracapsular) fractures are treated with a dynamic hip screw. In elderly people, osteoporosis is common and fracture occurs after a minor fall, therefore in such a patient with a fracture of the femoral neck the fracture is pathological. Fracture through a metastasis does occur but it is relatively uncommon occurrence at this site.

33 BCDE

Carotid body tumours, or chemodectomas, arise from paraganglionic neural crest cells and are richly supplied by chemoreceptors. Carotid body tumours arise in the wall of the carotid body, at the carotid bifurcation. They usually present with a lump in the neck which is mobile in a horizontal plane, or as a pulsatile mass. Baroreceptor problems may cause changes in blood pressure and syncope. Chronic exposure to low oxygen tension, such as encountered at high altitude, is known to increase the risk of chemodectoma. Angiography and duplex ultrasound are useful in the assessment of the condition.

34 CD

The incidence of this condition is 1 in 3500, the commonest form being a blind ending oesophagus with the trachea joining the lower bud from the stomach near the carina. Gas may be present in the bowel if there is a communication between the trachea and the remainder of the bowel. If there is a small distance between the ends of the oesophagus, a direct anastomosis can be fashioned safely.

With large gaps between the oesophageal ends, colonic interposition may be used to fashion a new conduit. A tracheo-oesophageal fistula is present in over 90% of cases of oesophageal atresia.

35 A

Although recurrent prostatitis may be treated with TURP, the results are disappointing and it is not an absolute indication. There is little correlation between residual volumes and renal impairment.

36 ABC

The spermatic cord contains:

3 fascial layers (external spermatic, cremasteric, internal spermatic).

3 arteries (testicular, cremasteric, vas deferens).

Other structures include: pampiniform plexus, vas deferens; and the genital branch of the genitofemoral nerve, sympathetic fibres and lymphatics. The ilioinguinal nerve enters the inguinal canal but not the spermatic cord.

37 CDE

The medial ligament of the ankle, otherwise known as the deltoid ligament, has two layers. The deep part is narrow and much shorter than the superficial part which is triangular in shape. The superficial part of the medial ligament is attached to the borders of the tibial malleolus, and has a continuous attachment from the medial tubercule of the talus along the edge of the sustentaculum tali and spring ligament to the tuberosity of the navicular bone. The lateral ligament consists of three separate bands, and it is this ligament which is usually damaged in inversion injuries (a sprain) of the ankle. The ligaments themselves cannot be seen on X-ray, although avulsion fractures may be detectable on X-ray.

38 BCDE

Postsplenectomy sepsis can present 20 years after splenectomy and carries a high mortality (50%). It is prevented by penicillin prophylaxis which should be lifelong. The micro-organisms most likely to lead to infection include pneumococcus, meningococcus and *H. influenzae.* Other infections include those due to *E. coli* and malaria.

39 BC

Testicular torsion is a surgical emergency that requires prompt diagnosis and urgent surgical treatment to prevent venous infarction and consequent necrosis of testis. Time should not be wasted by organising an ultrasound, which will add little to the management. During the operation, the untwisted testis is sutured to the tunica vaginalis or placed into a dartos pouch to prevent recurrence. Both testes should be secured since predisposition to torsion is usually bilateral. Maldescended testes are 30 times more likely to become malignant than normally descended testes. The risk of malignant change is also greater if there is a history of orchidopexy.

40 BCD

The IVC commences opposite the L5 vertebra. It runs on the right side of the aorta, upwards beyond the aortic opening of the diaphragm and extends to the central tendon of the diaphragm, which it pierces at the level of T8. The IVC lies behind the portal vein near the pancreas and bile duct, and forms the posterior wall of the epiploic foramen of Winslow. The right vein of the suprarenal gland is usually only a few millimetres long and enters the IVC directly. The left suprarenal vein is longer and enters the left renal vein.

41 CE

Transplanted kidneys are usually sited in an extraperitoneal position. A right donor kidney is more technically demanding to graft because of the short right renal vein. A living donor transplant has a higher survival benefit than a cadaveric transplant, equivalent to a 10% benefit at 5 years.

42 D

The processus vaginalis is a parietal peritoneal sac which passes through the internal ring of the inguinal canal in the fetus, but which is normally obliterated after birth except for a small part that becomes the tunica vaginalis of the testis. The testis descends through the canal as a retroperitoneal structure and is therefore outside and behind the processus vaginalis. In cases of a persistent processus vaginalis, indirect inguinal hernias can ensue.

43 BDE

The shoulder is the joint that dislocates most frequently, having an overall incidence of approximately 1.7%. More than 90% of shoulder dislocations are anterior with only approximately 3% being posterior. Inferior dislocations can occur but they are even more unusual. Injuries to the axillary nerve and brachial plexus are common and should be identified prior to reduction. An axillary nerve palsy occurs in between 9 and 18% of dislocations with weakness of the deltoid and numbness in the distribution of the regimental badge area on the lateral aspect of the upper arm. Spontaneous recovery following axillary nerve palsy is the norm. Brachial plexus injuries may be as high as 10%.

To confirm the diagnosis of a shoulder dislocation, anterior posterior and lateral scapula views are required. Anterior dislocations are usually obvious but the diagnosis of a posterior dislocation is often missed. Reduction is usually by closed manipulation.

44 DE

ERCP can be both diagnostic and therapeutic. It can be used to examine both the biliary tree and pancreatic duct. Biliary strictures and bile duct calculi can be identified. Sphincterotomy can be performed for intraductal biliary calculi and stents can be inserted to assist bile drainage, as in malignant obstruction.

45 BDE

The adductor canal (also known as the subsartorial or Hunter's canal) is a 15-cm long tunnel bounded by vastus medialis laterally, adductor longus and magnus posteriorly. The canal serves as a passage for the superficial femoral artery, femoral vein, saphenous nerve and the nerve to the vastus medialis to pass into the popliteal fossa. The adductor canal begins where the sartorius crosses over the adductor longus and ends at the adductor hiatus. The femoral artery gives off a descending genicular artery whilst in the adductor canal. The nerve to the tensor fascia lata is the superior gluteal nerve (L4–S1) which passes through the greater sciatic foramen.

46 AC

Pleomorphic adenoma, also known as mixed tumour, contains stromal and epithelial elements. It accounts for 60% of all parotid tumours. Although slow growing, it may be quite large at the time of presentation. Facial nerve palsy is a rare complication. The tumour is frequently multicentral and has no true capsule; therefore it may recur after surgery. The aim of surgery is complete excision of the tumour including a margin of normal parotid tissue. Radiotherapy has no substantial role in treatment.

47 ABCE

Faecal incontinence has a multitude of causes and these may be divided into trauma, colorectal disease, congenital abnormalities, neurological disease and miscellaneous conditions. Surgical trauma includes fissure surgery, haemorrhoidectomy, lateral sphincterotomy and anal stretch. Others include obstetric injuries. Inflammatory bowel disease and malignant tumours, haemorrhoids and rectal prolapse can themselves cause faecal incontinence. Congenital abnormalities include spina bifida and Hirschsprung's disease. Neurological disease includes cerebral disease (such as tumours, cerebrovascular accidents and trauma), while miscellaneous conditions include laxative abuse, faecal impaction and encopresis.

48 D

Ribs are narrow, flat, curved bones that form the thoracic cage. The rib has an angle at its posterior end. The costal groove is found on the inferior border of the ribs. The intercostal vessels and nerve run in this groove. Ribs typically articulate with their corresponding vertebra plus the one above it. The area just anterior to the angle is the weakest, therefore is the most likely to fracture in trauma.

49 ACD

Carcinoma of the gallbladder has a 90% association with gallstones and is the most common malignancy of the biliary tract. The finding of carcinoma of the gallbladder is often accidentally during cholecystectomy or incidentally at the time of histology. There is a very poor response to chemotherapy, with the 5-year survival rate approaching only 10%.

50 CE

The supraorbital nerve branches off its parent nerve (the frontal nerve) at the orbital margin, so strictly speaking it does not pass through the greater orbital fissure. The following pass through the superior orbital fissure: CN III, IV, VI, lacrimal, frontal, nasociliary nerves and the superior ophthalmic vein. The ophthalmic artery enters the orbit through the optic canal. The frontal nerve, along with the lacrimal and CN IV, enter the orbit outside the tendinous ring through the superior orbital fissure. The optic nerve is surrounded by all layers of the meninges, explaining the fundal changes seen in raised intracranial pressure. The superior branch of CN III supplies the levator palpebrae superioris muscle responsible for raising the eyelid.

51 BD

Colour Doppler is not 100% reliable, so if there is any suspicion of torsion of the testis then exploration must be carried out. Peak incidence is 14–18 years. Younger children are more likely to have a torted hydatid of Morgagni. Torsion of the testis is a surgical emergency. Most testes are viable for up to 4 hours after the onset of torsion. There are reports of viable testis for up to 72 hours, although this is more likely with intermittent torsion. Extravaginal torsion (torsion of the cord) occurs in utero or shortly after birth.

52 AC

The axillary artery commences at the lateral border of the first rib and continues as the subclavian artery. The axillary artery becomes the brachial artery at the inferior border of teres major. The axillary artery may be divided into three parts by the pectoralis minor. In its first part, it gives off the superior thoracic artery; in the second part, the thoracoacromial and lateral thoracic arteries; and in the third part, the subscapular, anterior and posterior circumflex arteries.

53 D

Supracondylar fractures of the humerus are likely to heal with an unsightly malunion unless a good position is achieved, as the medial epicondyle is pushed backwards and medially. Medial epicondylar avulsion occurs through a valgus force strain and causes stretching of the ulnar nerve and subsequent palsy. A pulled elbow is common in children under the age of 4 years and is caused by lifting the child up by its hands. The radial head can then slip partly out of the annular ligament. Non-union of a lateral condyle fracture will result in a valgus deformity stretching the ulnar nerve and, in rare instances, an ulnar nerve palsy.

54 BCDE

The right and left gastric arteries supply the lesser omentum as they lie between its two peritoneal layers. The free edge of the lesser omentum is attached to the first 2 cm of the first part of the duodenum below and the fissure of the ligamentum venosum above. The common hepatic duct is joined by the cystic duct to form the common bile duct in the free edge of the lesser omentum. The greater omentum is quite mobile.

55 D

Smoking appears protective against ulcerative colitis, but increases the risk of developing Crohn's disease and doubles the risk of postoperative recurrence. There is some evidence that the measles virus may have a causal relationship with Crohn's disease, but no definitive link has been established. When considering the extended family, 20–30% of patients with Crohn's disease have a positive family history. The risk of a child of a patient with Crohn's disease developing the disease is approximately 2%.

56 ACDE

Sjögren's syndrome manifests as dry eyes and dry mouth. It is associated with many immunological conditions, most commonly rheumatoid arthritis but also with SLE. It may occur alone in the absence of RA. Rheumatoid factor is usually present even in primary disease. Anti-Ro antibodies and circulating immune complexes are also found in the blood. The exocrine glands are infiltrated with lymphocytes and plasma cells, thereby causing their destruction and resulting in dry eyes and dry mouth. Frey's syndrome occurs after parotid surgery.

57 BCD

The subclavian artery is closely related to the brachial plexus, phrenic, vagus (and recurrent laryngeal nerve on the right side only). The stellate ganglion is deeper within the neck and the thoracic duct lies on the left side. The approach to the subclavian artery may be supraclavicular and involve removal or division of the clavicle, dissection of the scalenus anterior, pectoralis major and minor muscles.

58 ADE

'Hot' laparoscopic cholecystectomy can usually be safely performed in the first 72 hours, but only by an experienced surgeon as the risk of complications is greater. Acalculous cholecystitis may complicate trauma, sepsis and burns, but rarely occurs de novo. The HIDA scan would demonstrate a non-functioning gallbladder in a case of acute cholecystitis. A recognised but rare complication of acute cholecystitis is biliary peritonitis, due to gallbladder perforation.

59 ACDEF

Most of the anterior surface of the uterus is applied to the posterior surface of the bladder. Ureteric calculi are palpable through the posterior fornix, lateral to the cervix where the ureter passes under the uterine artery ('water under the bridge'). Lymphatic drainage of the medial part of the fallopian tubes and uterine fundus is via the lymphatics in the broad ligament to the superficial inguinal nodes. The main arterial supply of the uterus is from the uterine artery, a branch of the internal iliac. The round ligament is a gubernacular remnant.

60 ACDE

Parasympathetic fibres supply the main motor innervation of the bladder via the pelvic splanchnic nerves (S2–S4). Sympathetic fibres come from L1–L2 via the superior hypogastric and pelvic plexuses. The external sphincter contains skeletal muscle and is supplied by the perineal branch of the pudendal nerve (S2–S4). The obturator nerve, which is a branch of the lumbar plexus, is formed within the substance of the psoas major from the anterior divisions of the L2–L4 and supplies some parietal peritoneum and skin on the medial side of the thigh.

61 ADE

The 'important' cortical areas of the temporal lobe area are the auditory cortex and temporal association area (responsible for the recognition of auditory stimuli and integration with other modalities). Cerebral abscesses act as space-occupying lesions and produce focal neurological deficits. They may also cause meningitis, epilepsy and intracranial herniation.

62 ACD

Compartment syndrome is caused by increased pressure within the compartment(s) of a limb. If suspected, it must be treated aggressively. Measurement of intracompartmental pressures is sometimes useful. Compartment pressures should be less than 30 mmHg. If pressures are raised or there is a degree of clinical suspicion of a compartment syndrome, then open fasciotomy of all involved compartments must take place urgently. The main arterial supply to the extremity is not usually affected by the compartment syndrome and thus the hand or foot is warm and pink – unless, of course, the compartment syndrome is secondary to a reperfusion injury or if the blood pressure is low, for example after haemorrhage. Compartment syndrome may be seen in children, for example following 'minor' tibial shaft fractures or a supracondylar fracture of the humerus.

63 A

The superficial venous network (dorsal venous arch) on the dorsum of the hand drains partly into the cephalic vein just distal to the anatomical snuff-box. The cephalic vein then winds around onto the anterolateral aspect of the forearm. It runs in the upper arm lateral to the biceps in the deltopectoral groove and perforates the clavipectoral fascia to drain into the axillary vein. The axillary vein is formed by the union of the vena comitantes of the brachial artery and the basilic vein at the lower border of the teres major muscle.

64 CE

Ulcerative colitis is a mucosal inflammatory process which invariably involves the rectum and spreads in a proximal direction. In fulminant cases, the whole thickness of the bowel wall may be involved. Ulcerative colitis is confined to the rectum and distal sigmoid in 60% of cases. The cancer risk is greater in patients with a pancolitis and those presenting at a younger age. The exact risk varies from series to series but is approximately 1% at 10 years and 5% at 20 years. The presence of granulomas would strongly suggest a diagnosis of Crohn's disease.

65 ACDE

ESWL is contraindicated in pregnancy and in patients with aortic aneurysms where the aneurysm lies directly in the 'blast path'. Caution must be taken with patients who have pacemakers or those with clotting abnormalities. Steinstrasse (stone street) is a recognised complication of ESWL. It can be avoided if a ureteric stent is inserted before treatment, especially where the stone bulk exceeds 1.5 cm.

PRACTICE PAPER 1 – EMQ ANSWERS

Treatment of thyroid disease
66 A Carbimazole
67 B Propylthiouracil
68 C Radio-iodine

The first patient has Grave's disease, the treatment of which is medical. Carbimazole is the most widely used first-line agent in the UK. The most significant side-effect is agranulocytosis. Thus, regular blood tests are required. Propylthiouracil is used if the patient suffers sensitivity reactions to carbimazole.

Mild hyperthyroidism is common in pregnancy. If this requires treatment, antithyroid drugs are the most common first-line therapy. Propylthiouracil is used in pregnancy as it is more protein-bound and therefore less likely to cross the placenta. Close monitoring of T_3 and T_4 levels is required.

Previously, radio-iodine was only given to adults. It is now considered to be safe for all age groups as 40-year follow-up studies have shown no increased carcinogenic or sterility risk.

Shoulder pain
69 B Supraspinatus rupture
70 A Supraspinatus tendonitis

A complete tear of the supraspinatus tendon may occur after a long period of chronic tendonitis. Active abduction is impossible and attempting it produces a characteristic shrug; however, passive abduction is full and once the arm has been lifted to above a right angle the patient can keep it raised using the deltoid (abduction paradox).

Supraspinatus tendinitis usually occurs in patients <40 years of age who develop shoulder pain after vigorous/strenuous exercise. On active abduction the scapulohumeral rhythm is disturbed and pain is aggravated as the arm traverses an arc between 60 and 120°.

Low back pain
71 F Spondylolisthesis
72 B Muscle strain
73 D Osteoporotic collapse
74 G Discitis
75 E Metastatic disease

Spondylolisthesis commonly presents in the teenage years with pain and hamstring tightness. This is not the same as a limited straight-leg raise where the 'strain' is on the sciatic nerve.

Muscle strains are the most common cause of low back pain in fit, young adults particularly if there has been some 'unaccustomed' exercise. A slipped disc is more likely to be associated with radiation of the pain and symptoms of nerve root irritation.
88-year-olds often have osteoporosis and a simple fall can cause an osteoporotic fracture with collapse. As she is getting better, a more sinister explanation is unlikely.
In children who refuse to walk, a septic arthritis or osteomyelitis affecting the lower limbs must first be excluded; only then may a diagnosis of discitis be considered.
Although the man in scenario 75 is relatively young, his history of progressive pain radiating to the buttocks and cauda equina symptoms must raise the concern of a metastatic lesion.

Complications of hip surgery

76 C Urinary retention, male
77 A Death
78 E Wound infection without prophylaxis
79 D DVT, no prophylaxis
80 B Pulmonary embolus, no prophylaxis

Prophylaxis has had a marked impact on the reduction of deep wound infections and thrombotic complications. The risk of deep wound infection has dropped from 1–5% to <1% and the risk of a DVT from 60% to 15%. The risk of a PE in a patient on low-molecular-weight heparin is now 1–5%.

Anatomy of joints in the head and neck

81 D Cricothyroid
82 C Intervertebral disc
83 B Temporomandibular
84 A Atlanto-occipital

Rotatory movements at the cricothyroid joints tilt the thyroid cartilage forward, thereby elongating/tensing the vocal cords.
Intervertebral discs are secondary fibrocartilagenous joints allowing movement.
The axis of rotation of the mandible is not through the TMJ but through the lingula of the mandible. The movement is compound and comprises contemporaneous protraction onto the glenoid eminence with flexion.
Flexion of the head occurs at the atlanto-occipital joint.

Paediatric conditions

85 D Intussusception

86 A Pyloric stenosis

87 C Meckel's diverticulum

A sausage-shaped mass may be seen in intussusception or pyloric stenosis. However, bilious vomiting is not a feature of pyloric stenosis. Rectal bleeding with the production of 'redcurrant jelly' stools is seen in intussusception.

The patient in question 86 has the classical features of pyloric stenosis.

Meckel's diverticulum may give rise to rectal bleeding as 5% of cases have ectopic gastric mucosa.

Neonatal surgical diagnoses

88 A Hirschsprung's disease

89 G Exomphalos

90 H Mid-gut volvulus

91 B Oesophageal atresia

92 C Tracheo-oesophageal fistula

Hirschsprung's disease usually presents in the neonatal period with a history of delayed passage of meconium, abdominal distension and bile-stained vomiting. The infant may well be shocked with impending enterocolitis. Hirschsprung's disease is more common in children with Down's syndrome (trisomy 21). It can be differentiated postnatally from duodenal atresia in which there is passage of meconium, even in complete atresia.

Both gastroschisis and exomphalos are frequently diagnosed antenatally. In exomphalos, the liver is frequently outside the abdomen and the herniated organs are covered by an identifiable membrane.

Bile-stained vomiting in a previously well infant should raise the suspicion of a mid-gut volvulus.

A baby with oesophageal atresia is frequently born to a mother with a polyhydramnios. At birth the infant is unable to swallow even saliva, which froths through the mouth and nose.

Oesophageal atresia can occur with or without a tracheo-oesophageal fistula, which itself can occur in isolation. When an infant feeds, there may be aspiration of milk through the fistula into the lungs. Occasionally the infant may be several months old before the diagnosis is made.

Anatomy of abdominal vasculature

93 E Left renal vein
94 J Ileocolic artery
95 M Superior mesenteric artery
96 K Splenic artery

The left suprarenal gland drains into the left renal vein (along with the left gonadal vein).
The ileocolic artery supplies the caecum and appendix.
The superior mesenteric artery lies to the left of the vein, anterior to the uncinate process of the pancreas.
The short gastric branches of the splenic artery passing in the gastrosplenic ligament supply the fundus of the stomach.

Anatomy of the inguinal canal

97 D Floor
98 A Anterior wall
99 C Posterior wall
100 B Roof

Boundaries of the inguinal canal:

Floor:	Inguinal ligament (with lacunar ligament medially)
Anterior:	External oblique (with internal oblique laterally)
Posterior:	Transversalis fascia strengthened medially by conjoint tendon
Roof:	Lateral to medial – transversus abdominis, internal oblique, conjoint tendon

Infective and non-infective intestinal inflammation

101 B *Yersinia* enterocolitis
102 D Infective colitis
103 E Diversion colitis
104 A Amoebic dysentery
105 C Pseudomembranous colitis

Amoebic dysentery is typically associated with flask-shaped ulcers in the large bowel, caused by *Entamoeba histolytica*. The diamond-shaped ulcers have overhanging edges and a longitudinal axis at right angles to the colon.
Yersinia enterocolitis is associated with an acute ileitis with inflamed mesenteric lymph nodes. The terminal ileum and caecum are inflamed and oedematous, with superficial mucosal ulceration.
Pseudomembranous colitis is associated with characteristic yellow grey plaques on sigmoidoscopy. Infective colitis gives rise to features of oedema of the lamina propria and a predominant polymorphonuclear infiltrate.

This helps differentiation from other forms of colitis such as Crohn's disease or ulcerative colitis, which have both chronic and acute cells. Diversion colitis is thought to be due to a local butyrate deficiency, and may be treated with short-chain fatty acid solutions.

Jaundice

106 C Posthepatic jaundice
107 B Hepatic jaundice
108 A Prehepatic jaundice
109 B Hepatic jaundice
110 B Hepatic jaundice
111 B Hepatic jaundice
112 A Prehepatic jaundice
113 C Posthepatic jaundice
114 B Hepatic jaundice
115 A Prehepatic jaundice

Jaundice (icterus) is the yellow pigmentation of skin, sclera and mucosa due to a raised plasma bilirubin (>35 μmol/l). Pruritus is due to bile-salt deposition in the skin.

Prehepatic causes of jaundice include haemolytic anaemia and familial non-haemolytic hyperbilirubinaemia such as in Gilbert's and Rotor's syndromes.

Hepatic causes include acute viral or drug-induced (halothane, chlorpromazine) hepatitis, other hepatoxic substances (alcohol, carbon tetrachloride), cirrhosis, chronic active hepatitis, hepatic tumours, hydatid disease and liver abscesses.

Posthepatic causes include porta hepatis lymph nodes, sclerosing cholangitis, biliary atresia, bile duct carcinoma, pancreatic carcinoma and choledocholithiasis.

Colorectal surgery

116 F Abdominoperineal resection
117 E Subtotal colectomy
118 H Hartmann's procedure

The first case is of a man with a recurrence of his anal carcinoma. He has undergone chemoradiotherapy which has failed. The only treatment for his continued bleeding is surgery in the form of an abdominoperineal resection.

The second case is of a young woman with a flare-up of her ulcerative colitis, failed medical treatment and development of a toxic megacolon. In this instance, the surgical option is a subtotal colectomy with ileostomy, as she is at imminent risk of perforation. Her rectum is not excised, as this would increase the length of surgery and increase her morbidity. In addition, as she is young the possibility of a future ileoanal pouch should be left open to her.

The third case is of a man with a probable perforated sigmoid carcinoma and single metastasis to the liver. The carcinoma should be resected. A primary anastomosis in the presence of gross faecal contamination would be unwise. However, purulent peritonitis is itself not an absolute contraindication to a primary anastomosis. This should only be performed by an experienced surgeon and the majority would cover with a loop ileostomy.

Anatomy of the urogenital system

119 E Vas deferens
120 F Suspensory ligament of the ovary
121 C Urethra
122 H Perineal membrane
123 A Uterus
124 B Round ligament of the ovary
125 D Bladder

The vas deferens lies above the ureter, as the latter enters the bladder.

The ovarian vessels are transmitted by the suspensory ligament of the ovary (infundibulopelvic fold). This is the part of the broad ligament lateral to the attachment of the ovary.

Contraction of the internal sphincter of the male urethra prevents retrograde ejaculation into the bladder. After destruction of the sphincter at prostatectomy, ejaculation into the bladder occurs.

The perineal membrane supports the penis and is pierced by the urethra and dorsal vein of the penis.

The uterus is separated from the rectum by the pouch of Douglas. In males, the upper third of the rectum is completely surrounded by peritoneum, the middle third has the anterior half covered in peritoneum and the lower third has no peritoneal attachment. This anterior peritoneum sweeps forward over the top of the bladder, leaving only the fascia of Denonvillier between the male rectum and bladder/prostate.

The round ligament of the ovary is attached to the lateral wall of the uterus just below the isthmus of the fallopian tube. It is the fibrosed remnant of the gubernaculum.

The bladder intervenes between the uterus and pubic symphysis.

PRACTICE PAPER 2 – MCQ ANSWERS

1 BDE

Heberden's nodes occur in osteoarthritis and represent swollen distal interphalangeal joints. Rheumatoid arthritis is a symmetrical polyarthritis with early-morning stiffness and a raised ESR. The pathogenesis involves a sequence of synovitis, joint destruction and deformity. Typical X-ray features of rheumatoid arthritis are:

Early: soft tissue swelling, periarticular osteoporosis
Late: marginal bony erosions, narrowing of the articular space
Advanced: articular destruction and joint deformity.

2 ABC

Patients with bladder calculi usually present with irritative symptoms (frequency, urgency) rather than poor flow and hesitancy. A plain radiograph or ultrasound examination is required to make the diagnosis.

3 BCD

The medial wall, which separates the middle from the internal ear, contains the oval window and promontory. The promontory is the rounded projection of the first turn of the cochlea. Also medially, the internal auditory meatus carries the facial nerve. The floor is a thin bone separating the middle ear from the bulb of the jugular vein. Anteriorly, a thin bone wall separates the cavity from the internal carotid artery.

4 AB

Traumatic rupture of the oesophagus has a high morbidity and mortality. Extravasation of swallowed air results in mediastinal emphysema, and unchecked mediastinal soiling results in mediastinitis. A Gastrografin swallow is the diagnostic modality of choice. Boerhaave's syndrome refers to spontaneous lower oesophageal rupture during vomiting. When perforation is due to oesophagoscopy the tear is usually near the level of the cricoid cartilage, resulting from crushing against the cervical spine, which is often osteoarthritic.

5 DE

The palatine tonsil lies in the oropharynx, in a pit floored by the superior constrictor muscle through which CN IX passes. The tonsil is supplied by the tonsillar branch of the facial artery. Venous blood first drains into the tonsillar venous plexus, then into the pharyngeal venous plexus and thence into the external palatine vein (a bleeding point after tonsillectomy), or the facial and pharyngeal veins.

6 BDE

Long-standing massive splenomegaly is known to be caused by chronic malaria, chronic myeloid leukaemia, myelofibrosis, kala-azar and schistosomiasis. Chagas' disease causes oesophageal and gastrointestinal dilation. Hepatitis C is associated with cirrhosis of the liver, which may in turn produce splenomegaly. However, the splenomegaly is only moderate.

7 AFG

Keloid scars are more common on pigmented skin, burns, trauma wounds and those with a past history of keloid scars. There is excessive production and contraction of fibrous tissue. Greater success has been claimed for triamcinolone (steroid) injections which produce collagen lysis, whereas surgical excision may only result in a larger scar. Keloids occur on the dorsal areas of the body and over the face and deltopectoral region. The difference between keloid scarring and hypertrophic scarring is that the former heals by extending beyond the original boundary of incision, whereas the latter is a thickened scar within the initial incision.

8 ABE

Surgery for lymphoedema can be classified into reducing or bypass operations. In reducing operations, the lymphodematous subcutaneous tissue and skin are excised. In bypass operations, the sites of localised lymphatic obstruction are bypassed. Examples of reduction operations include Charles' and Homan's operations. Kinmonth's mesenteric bridge operation is an example of a bypass procedure.

9 ADE

Average-sized term infants require 150 ml/kg of formula feed per day. This will provide about 100 calories (419 J)/kg per day (the basic nutritional requirement). When a newborn infant undergoes surgery and requires intravenous fluids, it will require 100 ml of water/kg per day as well as 3 mmoles of sodium and 2 mmoles of potassium/kg per day. An infant undergoing surgery is under stress, and is at risk of hypoglycaemia. Therefore, a solution of 10% dextrose with 0.9% saline, to which is added 10 ml of potassium per 500 ml, will meet the infant's basic maintenance needs.

95% of term infants should pass meconium within the first 24 hours. Failure to do so might indicate a diagnosis of Hirschsprung's disease.

10 All true

The ischiorectal fossae, more accurately termed 'ischioanal fossae', are wedge-shaped fascia-lined spaces between the perianal skin and levator ani. Infection from one fossa may spread across the midline through the retrosphincteric space of the anococcygeal raphe posteriorly, but the anterior recesses extending above the perineal membrane remain separate. The base of each fossa is formed by skin and superficial fascia and may be easily incised to drain ischiorectal abscesses. The inferior rectal nerves and internal pudendal vessels are not usually damaged since they arch high in the roof.

11 BCE

The usual organism in acute septic arthritis of the knee is *Staphylococcus aureus*, but streptococci, gonococci and pneumococci are also seen. The joint is swollen, painful and inflamed, with an elevated WBC and ESR. Pus may also be aspirated. Systemic antibiotics should be started and irrigation of the joint carried out urgently. Complications include osteoarthritis in later years, or even total destruction of the joint. Locking is associated with meniscal tears. Weight-bearing is deferred for 4–6 weeks, but movement should occur prior to this.

12 BC

Gastric adenomas occur in 2–10% of patients with FAP, and duodenal adenomas in 30%. Hyperplastic gastric polyps are also common. Atrophic gastritis is not a recognised feature of the condition. Congenital hypertrophy of the retinal pigment epithelium is a common retinal abnormality occurring in FAP, but it is not pathognomonic of the condition. Uveitis is not a recognised feature of FAP. There is a 50–100 times increased risk of developing papillary thyroid cancer compared to the general population.

13 All false

The sciatic nerve appears in the gluteal region below the lower border of the piriformis muscle in the vast majority of cases, deep to the lower medial quadrant, and lateral to the inferior gluteal vessels. In its descent, it is separated from the capsule of the hip joint anteriorly by the obturator internus tendon, and by the gemelli muscles.

14 ABDE

The recurrent laryngeal nerves arise from the vagus. On the right, the recurrent laryngeal nerve winds around the subclavian artery; on the left, it winds around the aortic arch passing behind the ligamentum arteriosum. Both nerves run in a groove between the trachea and oesophagus and are closely related to the inferior thyroid artery.

15 ACE

Sigmoid volvulus is responsible for approximately 4% of all cases of intestinal obstruction in the UK. It is most common in the sixth and seventh decades, and in countries such as Africa. Predisposing factors include a redundant sigmoid colon and a long, narrow mesenteric attachment. Sigmoid volvulus is more common than caecal volvulus, and is associated with a long history of disordered bowel habit with chronic constipation and laxative abuse. The bowel twists in an anticlockwise direction and gives rise to the appearance of an omega loop on AXR (convexity lying away from site of obstruction). Circulation is not impaired until 1.5 twists have occurred.

16 ABD

Each renal artery usually divides into 5 segmental branches before entering the renal pelvis. It supplies the ureter and lies posterior to the renal vein, but anterior to the renal pelvis. After branching off the aorta, the renal artery passes in front of the IVC.

17 BDE

The peak incidence of acute appendicitis occurs during the 2nd and 3rd decades. It is rare at the extremes of age. The sequence of vomiting followed by abdominal pain should cast doubt over the diagnosis of acute appendicitis. An appendix mass is usually treated conservatively with antibiotics and percutaneous drainage of pus if indicated. An elective-interval appendectomy may be arranged after 8 weeks. It is important to investigate the >50-year-olds with barium enema to exclude a caecal carcinoma. Haematuria and diarrhoea are associated features of acute appendicitis.

18 CE

The abnormality in Hirschsprung's disease is aganglionosis of the large bowel. The abnormality starts at the anus and extends proximally. The male:female ratio is 5:1. The lumen of the aganglionic segment is narrowed, but the bowel proximal to this is grossly dilated. The aetiology of the enterocolitis that sometimes occurs in infants is obscure, but *Clostridium difficile* and *E. coli* endotoxin have been suggested.

19 BDE

A perforated duodenal ulcer is usually found on the anterior surface of the first part of the duodenum. Patients often present with a localised or more generalised peritonitis but silent perforations do occur, especially in elderly women. These may be treated conservatively. The operation of choice is patching with greater omentum loosely tied over the perforation. In cases of massive perforation, a partial gastrectomy may be required as it may be impossible to bring the edges of the duodenum safely together.

20 BCE

In Western populations, the approximate prevalence of Crohn's disease is 1 in 1500, and that of ulcerative colitis is 1 in 1000. The prevalence of IBD is the same in different social classes. There is, however, an increased incidence of both ulcerative colitis and Crohn's disease in Jews living outside Israel, suggesting a multifactorial aetiology involving environmental and genetic mechanisms.

21 ACE

The major arterial supply to the ureter is (from superior to inferior): the renal artery, the gonadal artery and the superior vesical artery. The blood supply to the ureter is reinforced at intervals by small branches of the lumbar arteries. The ureter lies posterior to the gonadal vessels and vas, but descends anterior to the psoas muscle and the bifurcation of the common iliac artery.

22 ABDE

The popliteus tendon penetrates the capsule and is covered by synovial membrane. The suprapatellar bursa, although developing as an isolated cavity, later fuses with the joint space. The iliotibial tract is attached to a smooth round facet on the anterolateral aspect of the lateral condyle of the tibia. The middle geniculate artery pierces the joint capsule to supply it and the cruciate ligaments. Flexion occurs in the upper compartment and rotation in the lower compartment of the knee.

23 A

Colorectal cancer causes 19,000 deaths per annum in the UK (OPCS, 1995). It is second only to lung cancer in importance as a cause of cancer death, with figures approaching 12% (breast cancer accounts for 9% of cancer deaths).

Colon cancer occurs with an equal incidence in men and women, but rectal cancer is more common in men. The extremely low incidence of colorectal carcinoma in Africa is thought to be related to dietary fibre. Having a single relative who has had colorectal cancer will increase an individual's risk to 1 in 17.

24 BD

Graves' disease accounts for about 90% of cases of thyrotoxicosis. It is more common in women (10:1) and is caused by thyroid-stimulating immunoglobulins. Thyrotoxicosis is a multisystem disease affecting all organs.

General:	weight loss, increased appetite, fever, sweating, heat intolerance
CVS:	palpitations, angina, CVS failure, atrial fibrillation
Neurological:	tremor, psychosis, proximal myopathy, myasthenia, choreoathetosis
GIT:	vomiting, diarrhoea, steatorrhoea
Skin:	hyperpigmentation, acropachy, spider naevi, palmar erythema, pretibial myxoedema
Bones:	osteoporosis
Eyes:	lid lag and lid retraction; 50% of Graves' sufferers have ophthalmic changes, e.g. exophthalmos, ophthalmoplegia, chemosis (conjunctival oedema)
Reproductive:	oligomenorrhoea, gynaecomastia.

25 CDE

Congenital dislocation of the hip is part of a spectrum of hip abnormalities. It occurs in 5–20/1000 live births – girls:boys 7:1 with the left hip affected more than the right. 1 in 5 cases is bilateral. It tends to be more common for babies delivered in the breech position. Ultrasound will demonstrate the shape of the cartilaginous socket and position of the femoral head. It may present in adults (30–40 years of age) with increasing discomfort in the hip, difficulty walking and backache. Ortolani's and Barlow's tests can be used in screening and diagnosis.

26 ABD

Neurological signs develop as there may be involvement of the vertebral, carotid or spinal vessels. Control of the blood pressure is the most important factor as over 50% of patients are hypertensive. A CT scan can diagnose an aortic dissection in 85% of cases. Transoesophageal echo or MRI are alternatives. An aortogram still remains the 'gold standard' investigation.

27 BCD

The trigeminal (V) nerve has sensory fibres to the greater part of the skin of the face, mucous membranes of the mouth, nose and paranasal air sinuses. It provides motor innervation to the muscles of mastication (temporalis, masseter, pterygoid). The buccinator muscle is supplied by the facial nerve. The angle of the mandible is supplied by the great auricular nerve (C2–C3).

28 CDE

The gold standard treatment of anal fissure is still lateral sphincterotomy (division of the internal anal sphincter). GTN is effective in the treatment of anal fissure, but it heals only 40–60% of chronic anal fissures and recurrence rates are considerable. Chronic anal fissure may be treated by diltiazem (calcium antagonist), botulinum toxin or an advancement flap.

29 ABC

Circumcision in infancy is associated with an extremely low risk of developing penile cancer in adult life. There is no proven association between prostatic cancer and vasectomy.

30 BD

Cervical rib is present in about 0.5% of the population, of which 60% are symptomatic. Symptoms due to the presence of a cervical rib depend on the structure it is compressing. Neurological symptoms are the most common presentation, usually compression of the C8 and T1 nerve roots cause pain and paraesthesia on the ulnar aspect of the arm and forearm and wasting of the small muscles of the hand. Vascular changes are seen less often. The arm can become swollen as a result of venous compression. Compression of the subclavian artery can lead to thrombus formation, emboli, ischaemic changes and even gangrene.

31 BD

Secondary haemorrhage occurs 5–10 days postoperatively. It is due to local sepsis, dislodgement of clot/sloughing or ligature erosion. This phenomenon is commonly seen in patients undergoing TURP. Anticoagulation may cause bleeding problems, but these are not classified as secondary haemorrhage.

32 BCE

Raynaud's syndrome can be idiopathic (Raynaud's disease) or secondary to an underlying cause (Raynaud's phenomenon). It is caused by vasospasm of the arterioles of the distal limbs after exposure to cold or emotional stimuli. There is characteristic colour change, pale → blue → red. Other causes of Raynaud's syndrome include the use of vibrating tools, systemic lupus erythematosus, scleroderma, trauma and atherosclerosis. Treatment options include keeping the limb warm, cessation of smoking, vasodilators (nifedipine), prostacyclin and cervical sympathectomy.

33 ACDE

Anorectal lesions associated with HIV-infected patients include: Kaposi's sarcoma; rectal ulceration; lymphoma; neurofibromas; anal fissure; anal fistula; perirectal abscess; squamous-cell carcinoma; and condylomata acuminata. Apocrine hydrocystoma is a rare apocrine tumour not directly unrelated to HIV.

34 All true

The base of the bladder is its posterior surface and is triangular. On the base of the bladder in the male, the vas deferens lies uppermost and loops medially over the ureters ('water under the bridge') which separate the seminal vesicle from the vas. In the female, the cervix and anterior vaginal wall are attached to the base of the bladder.

35 BC

A reduced serum calcium level causes an increase in PTH release. PTH increases the serum calcium level by acting on the kidney, bone and gut (indirectly). It causes increased renal reabsorption of calcium and increased conversion of vitamin D to 1,25-DHCC. In turn, 1,25-DHCC stimulates the intestinal absorption of calcium. Osteoclasts are also activated to increase bone resorption and so raise calcium levels.

36

The posterior relations of the right kidney are the diaphragm, quadratus lumborum, psoas, transversus abdominis, the 12th rib on the right and the 11th and 12th ribs on the left. Furthermore, the posterior recess of the pleura lies posteriorly as does the subcostal vein, artery and nerve (T12), and the ilioinguinal (L1) and iliohypogastric (L1) nerves. The suprarenal gland lies superomedial to the kidney.

37 B

The amount of blood lost from the GI tract is normally between 0.5 and 1.5 ml/day. This amount is typically not detected by occult blood tests. Occult blood is commonly detected in the stool by FOB tests when there is no clinical evidence of bleeding or iron deficiency. Guaiac-based FOB tests make use of the pseudoperoxidase activity of haemoglobin – guaiac turns blue after oxidation. Guaiac-based tests are generally best at detecting large distal lesions. Faecal rehydration markedly raises the sensitivity of the test but reduces its specificity. Whilst the dark-green or black appearance of iron in the stool can be confused with the typical blue appearance of a positive guaiac-based test, iron does not per se cause a positive reaction.

38 AB

The thyroid gland has a definite fine capsule, which allows a capsular dissection to preserve the recurrent laryngeal nerves. The superior parathyroid glands are more constant in position than the inferior. Because of their embryological migration, the inferior glands may be situated among the pretracheal lymph nodes or in the thymus as far as 10 cm from the thyroid. The middle thyroid veins are the least constant of the thyroid veins. The superior veins drain into the internal jugular vein; the inferior veins are very constant and drain into the brachiocephalic veins; and the middle veins are very variable and often multiple. Unilateral recurrent laryngeal nerve section results in the ipsilateral vocal cord lying motionless in the mid or cadaveric position. The voice is hoarse and weak. If both recurrent laryngeal nerves are divided then the glottic space is narrowed and stridor develops.

39 A

Infantile hypertrophic pyloric stenosis is a very common condition occurring in 3–5:1000 live births. The vomiting is typically effortless and forceful (projectile) and is not bile-stained as the intestinal obstruction is proximal to the ampulla of Vater. There is a well-recognised familial association. Babies born prematurely may develop pyloric stenosis. Although a test feed is helpful in palpation of the pyloric olive, it is equally possible to feel it whilst the infant is asleep, or at rest quietly sucking on a dummy. Abdominal ultrasound is routinely used to make the diagnosis of pyloric stenosis.

40 ABD

Tamsulosin and alfuzosin are alpha-blockers which relax the smooth muscle of the prostate and bladder neck. Tolterodine is an anticholinergic used in the treatment of detrusor instability. It may precipitate urinary retention. Finasteride is a 5α-reductase inhibitor which reduces prostate size. Goserelin is used in the treatment of prostate cancer.

41 ABE

In Horner's syndrome there is: ptosis, pupillary constriction and occasional enophthalmos; and dryness and flushing of the skin of the head and neck. The sympathetic supply to the lungs is preserved as this originates below the lesion directly from the T1–4. ganglia of the sympathetic chain. Sympathetic fibres pass to the arm via grey rami from the middle and inferior cervical sympathetic ganglia through all roots of the brachial plexus.

42 BCDF

The most common defect is the posterolateral or Bochdalek hernia. The anteromedial defect of Morgagni may not present till adult life. 80% of hernias occur on the left and 1% are bilateral. Herniation of bowel into the thorax causes lung compression and hypoplasia, presenting with neonatal respiratory distress and apparent dextrocardia. It is associated with other congenital defects in 50% of cases. Immediate nasogastric intubation and suction to decompress the bowel and stomach in the chest and intubation is required to stabilise the patient prior to surgery. There have been some successful attempts at repair in utero.

43 AC

This condition occurs at the age of 12–16 years with a male preponderance, and almost always coincides with the pubertal growth spurt. It is more common on the left than the right. The slip leads to an externally rotated leg and coxa vara. Complications include slipping of the opposite hip (20%), avascular necrosis (usually iatrogenic) and articular chondrolysis. Slipping is usually due to a number of small episodes rather than one sudden slip.

44 AB

Most abdominal aortic aneurysms are caused by atherosclerosis. *Salmonella* is the commonest cause of mycotic aneurysms. 98% of aneurysms are infrarenal. The 5-year rupture rate is 9% for aneurysms measuring <4.5 cm in diameter, 35% for aneurysm measuring 4.5–7 cm and 75% for aneurysms >7 cm in diameter.

45 BCDE

The trachea commences just below the cricoid cartilage (at the level of C6). Within the thorax and on the right, the trachea is in contact with the pleura, vagus and subclavian artery. On its left, the trachea is in contact with the left recurrent laryngeal nerve, aortic arch and left common carotid and subclavian arteries. The trachea ends at the upper border of T5 where it bifurcates.

46 ABD

Primary or spontaneous bacterial peritonitis is usually caused by the haematogenous spread of a single bacterium, most commonly a Gram-negative bacillus such as *E. coli*. There is an increased incidence of primary peritonitis in cirrhosis, ascites and nephrosis. The ascitic fluid has an increased white cell count. Signs may be obscured in the presence of pre-existing ascites.

47 BDE

Carcinoid tumours occur in the vermiform appendix (40%), small intestine (mainly ileum) (20%), large bowel (mainly rectum) (20%), lung and bronchus (10%) and other sites (10%). Most carcinoids of the appendix and rectum are benign and are incidental findings.

48 AE

The clinical features of seminoma include testicular pain, scrotal mass, secondary hydrocele, lymphadenopathy, gynaecomastia and symptoms due to metastases. Orchidectomy through an inguinal approach usually confirms the diagnosis of testicular cancer. The suspicion of testicular cancer is a contraindication to fine needle aspiration cytology (FNAC) and cone biopsy. Such investigations carry the risk of dissemination along the needle track and scrotal wall disease, which is difficult to control. The tumour is sensitive to radiotherapy and chemotherapy (carboplatin and etoposide).

49 ABD

Hydatid disease of the liver occurs when humans ingest the hexacanth embryos of the dog tapeworm *Echinococcus granulosus* or *E. multilocularis*. The embryos hatch in the duodenum and penetrate the intestinal wall to enter the portal system where they are carried to the liver. Further dissemination to the lung may occur. Rupture of hydatid cysts may cause jaundice and peritonitis. An eosinophilia is the abnormality seen in a peripheral blood film. Treatment is to excise the cyst if possible by first sterilising the cyst with formalin or alcohol. Medical treatment involves prolonged usage of albendazole.

50 All false

The prostate is an inverted cone, so it has a base in contact with the bladder neck above it and an apex lying against the urogenital diaphragm below it. The seminal vesicles drain into the vas deferens posterior to the bladder to form the common ejaculatory ducts, which pierce the prostate and empty into the prostatic urethra. The prostatic venous plexus lies outside the capsule and thus 'shelling' of the prostate from inside the capsule is a relatively avascular procedure. The prostate is separated from the rectum by the rectovesical fascia (of Denonvilliers).

51 ABCE

The pituitary sits in the sella turcica of the sphenoid. It is covered by the diaphragma sellae (fold of dura) which separates it from the optic chiasma above. There is an opening in the diaphragma for the pituitary stalk. The cavernous sinuses are found laterally and the sphenoid sinuses inferiorly.

52 C

The lateral malleolus is grooved by the peroneus brevis tendon; the medial malleolus by the tibialis posterior tendon. The superficial part of the deltoid ligament is attached to the sustentaculum tali of the calcaneus. Posterior to the medial malleolus, the tibial nerve lies posterior to the posterior tibial artery; the two lying between the flexor hallucis longus tendons posteriorly, and the flexor digitorum longus tendons anteriorly.

53 ACD

A below-knee amputation may be fashioned using a long posterior flap or a skew flap. Early physiotherapy, with mobilisation of the stump, is advocated to prevent contractures and stiffness. The stump must heal adequately before considering a prosthesis. After at least 6 weeks a PAMAID may be used. The stump does continue to shrink over the subsequent months, hence early fitting may need to be adjusted later on.

54 DE

When performing a right hemicolectomy, the gonadal vessels are encountered first and then the second part of the duodenum and right ureter. It is wise to clearly identify the ureter, although formal dissection and display is not always needed.

55 ACD

Exomphalos is associated with other abnormalities in about 40% cases. Syndromes include Beckwith–Wiedemann, Edwards and Patau. Respiratory distress may occur secondary to compression of the diaphragm. An omphalocele is a sac of fused amniotic membrane and peritoneum. In contrast, an exomphalos is due to herniation into the umbilical cord of gut contents. This may include viscera such as liver, spleen and bowel.

56 BCD

70–80% of pancreatic carcinomas arise in the head, neck or uncinate process. CT usually gives more information than ultrasound. Endoscopic ultrasound is being increasingly used for the assessment of pancreatic carcinoma. Features suggestive of irresectability include hepatic or lymph node metastases, ascites and invasion of the superior mesenteric vessels, portal vein and IVC. Typical radiological features on ERCP include localised stricturing of the main pancreatic and bile ducts, known as the 'double-duct' sign.

57 BC

The pharyngotympanic tube drains the middle ear into the nasopharynx by piercing the pharyngobasilar fascia. The cartilaginous part gives attachment to the tensor veli palatini muscle. It opens on swallowing under the action of the salpingopharyngeus and tensor palati muscles, and is obstructed by an enlarging pharyngeal tonsil (adenoids).

58 ACDEF

Most of the anterior surface of the uterus is applied to the posterior surface of the bladder. Ureteric calculi are palpable through the posterior fornix, lateral to the cervix where the ureter passes under the uterine artery ('water under the bridge'). Lymphatic drainage of the medial part of the fallopian tubes and uterine fundus is via the lymphatics in the broad ligament to the superficial inguinal nodes. The main arterial supply of the uterus is from the uterine artery, a branch of the internal iliac. The round ligament is a gubernacular remnant.

59 BCD

The blood supply to the scaphoid enters distally, thus in displaced fractures the proximal pole may be rendered avascular. Displaced scaphoid fractures are best treated by open reduction and internal fixation. Fractures of the scaphoid occur predominantly in young men and are associated with tenderness in the anatomical snuffbox. Most fractures of the scaphoid are treated by a below-elbow cast that includes the thumb.

60 A

Intussusception is more common in the summer months. No identifiable cause is found in 10% of patients. A Peyer's patch is the pathological lead-point in 75% of cases. The advancing inner segment is the intussusceptum, the outer the intussuscipiens. Classical 'redcurrant jelly stools' are seen in 20% of cases and are a late sign of intestinal ischaemia. Absence of viscera in the right lower quadrant on abdominal X-ray (Dances sign – 'feeling of emptiness') is seen in 15% of patients. Hydrostatic reduction after resuscitation and antibiotics should be tried unless there is peritonitis, pneumoperitoneum or septic shock. A flow of barium or Gastrografin into the terminal ileum indicates successful reduction. Air enemas are used in many units as an alternative. A right transverse supraumbilical incision is generally used; and after reduction, the appendix is removed. The risk of recurrence is 2–10%.

61 ABDE

Obstructive jaundice per se does not carry an increased risk of DVT, but if this is due to malignancy (e.g. carcinoma of the head of pancreas) then the risk is increased. Renal failure has a strong association with obstructive jaundice and is known to lead to the hepatorenal syndrome. There is an increased risk of wound dehiscence and incisional hernia in jaundiced patients. Due to impaired absorption of vitamin K and decreased production of clotting factors, the likelihood of a wound haematoma increases. The role of jaundice in impairing wound healing is probably multifactorial.

62 ABD

The facial nerve gives off a branch to the stapedius before it enters the stylomastoid foramen. The buccinator is supplied by the buccal branches of the facial nerve. The medial (and lateral) pterygoid is supplied by the mandibular division of the trigeminal nerve. The parasympathetic supply to the lacrimal gland is from the secretomotor fibres from the superior salivatory nucleus travelling in the intermediate and greater petrosal nerves and relaying in the pterygopalatine ganglion. The parasympathetic supply to the parotid gland is from the inferior salivatory nucleus via the tympanic and lesser petrosal branches of the glossopharyngeal nerve that project to the otic ganglion (preganglionic). Postganglionic fibres pass from the otic ganglion to the parotid via the auriculotemporal nerve.

63 B

Paget's disease causes enlargement and thickening of bone. However, the bone itself is brittle due to its abnormal internal architecture. Paget's disease mainly affects the tibia (bow-leg deformity) and pelvis; other sites include the femur, skull, spine (kyphosis) and clavicle. Both sexes are equally affected and Paget's disease usually presents after 50 years of age. Cranial nerves may be compressed due to skull enlargement (VII, VIII, V). The alkaline phosphatase level is raised and this is used as a marker for disease activity. Malignant change occurs in about 1% of cases. In rare instances, the prolonged increased blood flow to bone can lead to high-output cardiac failure.

64 A

Worthwhile benefit from surgery has only been demonstrated in patients with severe carotid (>70%) stenosis who have recently become symptomatic. Most surgeons would consider a large completed stroke as a contraindication for surgery.

65 E

Indirect inguinal hernias enter through the internal inguinal ring lateral to the inferior epigastric vessels. Direct inguinal hernias usually emerge through the medial aspect of the posterior wall of the inguinal canal. Sliding hernias may have the caecum, sigmoid or bladder forming part of the wall of the sac. Femoral hernias are more common in females, but, overall, inguinal hernias are more common than femoral hernias in women.

PRACTICE PAPER 2 – EMQ ANSWERS

Spinal pathology

66 A Acute disc prolapse

67 C TB of spine

Pain on hip extension represents a positive femoral stretch (L2, 3, 4). Only 5% of disc prolapses occur above L4–5. An acute disc prolapse will cause a scoliosis due to muscle spasm.

Scheuermann's disease is a condition of unknown cause affecting 1% of the population and often associated with a kyphosis. There is avascular necrosis of the ring apophyses and disc herniation through the endplate. It may be associated with excessive mechanical stress or endocrine abnormalities.

TB of the spine should always be suspected in patients from the Asian subcontinent. Note that the incidence of TB is increasing in the UK.

Nerve damage

68 D Neurapraxia of the common peroneal nerve

69 C Neurapraxia of the median nerve

70 H Neurotmesis of the medial nerve

71 A Horner's syndrome

72 F Sciatic nerve injury

The peroneal nerve is very susceptible to pressure, and thus may result in a neurapraxia. Following a supracondylar fracture of a child's humerus, a neurapraxia of the median nerve is the most common neurological lesion but damage to the ulnar nerve is also not uncommon.

If a surgical procedure is complicated by nerve injury, a transection (neurotmesis) must be considered – especially if the nerve has not been visualised.

A flail upper limb suggests a brachial plexus lesion, which might well be associated with Horner's syndrome if the sympathetic chain is involved.

During a hip replacement, two forms of nerve injury are well documented: direct damage to the sciatic nerve at the level of the hip joint (more common); and pressure on the peroneal nerve at the neck of the fibula. During a posterior approach to the hip, the sciatic nerve is in particular danger.

Knee injuries

73 F Tibial plateau fracture
74 C Patellar fracture
75 A Injury to the medial meniscus
76 B Anterior cruciate rupture
77 E Medial ligament rupture

A valgus force to the knee produced by a car bumper is likely to result in bony damage (a tibial plateau fracture), whilst a similarly directed force during a game of football is more likely to lead to rupture of the medial collateral ligament. Complete rupture of this ligament would lead to gross instability on weight-bearing at the time of injury. As the joint is disrupted, no discrete effusion is seen, although the area may be swollen and bruised. Swelling due to a medial meniscal injury usually takes some hours to become apparent. However, an anterior cruciate ligament rupture with the classical 'pop' produces a rapid haemarthrosis.

Paediatric newborn GI disorders

78 D Duodenal atresia
79 B Intussusception
80 A Hirschsprung's disease

A child with a scaphoid abdomen and bilious vomiting should be suspected of having duodenal atresia. Symptoms usually occur in the first few hours of life. The diagnosis may be made by injecting 30 ml of air via a nasogastric tube and taking a radiograph. This is not to be confused with the persistent vomiting of hypertrophic pyloric stenosis, which is not bile-stained and presents at 6 weeks.

A child with an abdominal mass, distension, passing meconium for 3 days and now passing blood, should be suspected of having an intussusception. It is only late in the disease that bleeding per rectum becomes a feature, suggesting mucosal necrosis.

Meconium ileus tends to present with a distended abdomen and bilious vomiting with no passage of meconium. The rectum is characteristically empty. 1:15,000 newborns have a distal small bowel obstruction secondary to abnormally bulky viscid meconium. 90% of these infants will have cystic fibrosis.

Hirschsprung's disease is the most common cause of intestinal obstruction in a newborn and affects 1:5000 children. Typically, there is delay in passing meconium beyond the first 24 hours of life with abdominal distension and bilious vomiting. Patients with Hirschsprung's disease may present after the neonatal period with chronic constipation or partial large bowel obstruction.

Thyroid disease

81 A Subtotal thyroidectomy
82 C Total thyroidectomy
83 C Total thyroidectomy

In case 81, subtotal thyroidectomy optimises the control of thyrotoxicosis whilst minimising complications.

Lymphoma of the thyroid is treated by surgery followed by radiotherapy to the neck and mediastinum.

Indications for thyroid surgery are:

carcinoma
compression (of trachea)/retrosternal extension
cosmesis
failed medical treatment

Parathyroid glands

84 B Superior parathyroid glands
85 B Superior parathyroid glands
86 A Inferior parathyroid glands
87 A Inferior parathyroid glands
88 B Superior parathyroid glands
89 A Inferior parathyroid glands

The inferior parathyroid glands, along with the thymus, are derived from the third branchial pouch. The superior parathyroid glands are derived from the fourth branchial pouch. The inferior glands are usually adjacent to the lower pole of the thyroid gland, but may lie anywhere from the mandible to the anterior mediastinum: 20% lie on or within the suprasternal portion of the thymus. The superior glands are normally found adjacent to the inferior thyroid artery just after it has started to branch, adjacent to the cricothyroid notch, and close to the recurrent laryngeal nerve. Overall, supernumerary glands occur in approximately 5% of the population.

Lymphatic drainage

90 B Para-aortic lymph nodes
91 D Superficial inguinal lymph nodes
92 D Superficial inguinal lymph nodes
93 A Internal iliac lymph nodes
94 A Internal iliac lymph nodes
95 D Superficial inguinal lymph nodes

The lymphatic drainage of an organ follows its arterial blood supply. For this reason the testicles will drain to the para-aortic lymph nodes, and not the inguinal nodes as would be expected from their location.

The anal canal derives from the hindgut (columnar epithelium) above and proctodeum (stratified squamous epithelium) below. Blood supply is therefore from the superior rectal branch of the inferior mesenteric artery above. Tumours arising here will spread to the para-aortic nodes. Blood supply to the inferior canal comes from the inferior rectal artery (a branch of the internal iliac artery), and therefore tumours will spread to the inguinal lymph nodes.

Anterior abdominal wall

96 G Below and lateral to the pubic tubercle
97 A Transpyloric plane
98 K 10th rib

The external ring of the femoral canal lies below and lateral to the pubic tubercle.

The spinal cord terminates in the transpyloric plane at the lower border of the L1 vertebra. The transpyloric plane of Addison lies halfway between the suprasternal notch and the pubic crest. At this level the pylorus, pancreatic neck, duodenal jejunal flexure (ligament of Treitz), fundus of the gallbladder, 9th costal cartilage, hilum of each kidney and the coeliac trunk may be seen.

The spleen lies on the left 9th, 10th and 11th ribs, posteriorly.

The L5 vertebral body lies in the transtubercular plane.

Hernias

99 A Epigastric hernia
100 C Obturator hernia
101 E Gluteal hernia

Epigastric hernias are often painful and may be multiple. Treatment is by suturing the defect in the linea alba.

Obturator hernias may present in old women as a cause of medial thigh pain. Obturator hernias are often difficult to diagnose and may only be found at the time of surgery for small bowel obstruction.

Surgical investigations

102 B Abdominal CT scan

103 F Barium enema (double-contrast)

104 D ERCP

105 D ERCP

Hepatic hydatid disease characteristically results in complex cysts with septation and daughter cysts, and is best seen on CT. Double-contrast barium enema is the most precise method of demonstrating the presence and extent of uncomplicated diverticular disease. Colonoscopy carries a high risk of complication in patients with diverticular disease.

ERCP defines ductal anatomical detail well, and may reveal the 'chain of lakes' of sclerosing cholangitis. Ultrasound may fail to show ductal dilatation or common duct stones. ERCP would provide a more definitive diagnosis and allow therapeutic manoeuvres for choledocholithiasis.

Abdominal pain investigations – diagnostic

106 C Erect chest X-ray

107 D Supine abdominal X-ray

108 C Erect chest X-ray

The first case is most likely to be a perforated duodenal ulcer and an erect CXR would be the best investigation.

The most likely diagnosis in the second patient would be a sigmoid volvulus and the supine AXR would show an omega loop.

The most likely diagnosis in the third patient is again a perforated peptic ulcer and an erect CXR would be most appropriate. Air is seen under the diaphragm in 90% of cases.

Anatomy of the posterior abdominal wall

109 H Superior rectal artery

110 C Lumbar plexus

111 A Kidney

112 G Bare area of the liver

The superior rectal artery (a branch of the inferior mesenteric artery) lies medial to the left ureter throughout its course.

The lumbar plexus is embedded in the psoas major muscle.

The kidney lies anterior to the subcostal vessels and nerve on each side.

The bare area of the liver contacts the right suprarenal gland.

Renal physiology
113 A Distal convoluted tubule
114 B Proximal convoluted tubule
115 B Proximal convoluted tubule
116 C Descending limb of loop of Henle
Sodium moves by co-transport or exchange from the tubular lumen into the tubular epithelial cells down its concentration gradient, and is actively pumped from these cells in to the interstitial space. Sodium is mostly absorbed in the proximal convoluted tubule (70%). Glucose reabsorption occurs in association with sodium in the early portion of the proximal convoluted tubule.
Facultative potassium control is in the distal convoluted tubule via the Na^+/K^+-ATPase pump, regulated by aldosterone.
The descending loop of Henle is permeable to water.

Pelvic vasculature
117 G Internal iliac artery
118 C Gonadal veins
119 A Superior gluteal artery
120 H Uterine artery
The ureter enters the pelvis by crossing anterior to the bifurcation of the common iliac artery and accompanies the internal iliac artery as far as its bifurcation into anterior and posterior divisions.
The middle third of the ureters are supplied by the gonadal arteries and drained by the gonadal veins.
The superior gluteal artery is the largest branch of the posterior division of the internal iliac artery.
The uterine artery runs in the base of the broad ligament. The condensation of connective tissue around the uterine vessels forms the transverse cervical ligament attaching the cervix to the lateral pelvic wall, thereby stabilising the uterus.

5-year graft patency rates
121 A Reversed vein femoropopliteal graft
122 E Femoral–femoral crossover graft
123 D Axillofemoral graft
124 B Femoropopliteal PTFE graft patency (below knee)
125 C Aortobifemoral graft
Patency rates are related to the force and volume of the inflow and the run-off away from the graft. If the run-off is poor then blood that passes into the graft will have nowhere to go, and flow will therefore be greatly reduced so leading to graft occlusion and failure. Synthetic grafts used below the inguinal ligament are vastly inferior to vein grafts.

INDEX

Locators are in the form chapter number.question/answer number. Thus 2.6 refers to chapter 2 question 6 and P1.93 to practice paper 1 question 93.

PASTEST COURSES

PASTEST: the key to exam success, the key to your future.
PasTest is dedicated to helping doctors to pass their professional examinations. We have 30 years of specialist experience in medical education and over 3000 doctors attend our revision courses each year.

Experienced lecturers:
Many of our lecturers are also examiners and teach in a lively and interesting way in order to:

- ✔ reflect current trends in exams
- ✔ give plenty of mock exam practice
- ✔ provide valuable advice on exam technique

Outstanding accelerated learning:
Our up-to-date and relevant course material includes MCQs, colour slides, X-rays, ECGs, EEGs, clinical cases, data interpretations, mock exams, vivas and extensive course notes which provide:

- ✔ hundreds of high quality questions with detailed answers and explanations
- ✔ succinct notes, diagrams and charts

Personal attention:
Active participation is encouraged on these courses, so in order to give personal tuition and to answer individual questions our course numbers are limited.
Book early to avoid disappointment.

Choice of courses:
PasTest has developed a wide range of high quality interactive courses in different cities around the UK to suit your individual needs.

What other candidates have said about our courses:
'Absolutely brilliant – I would not have passed without it! Thank you.'
Dr Charitha Rajapakse, London.
'Excellent, enjoyable, extremely hard work but worth every penny.'
Dr Helen Binns, Oxford.

For further details contact:

PasTest Ltd, Egerton Court, Parkgate Estate
Knutsford, Cheshire WA16 8DX, UK.

Telephone: 01565 752000 Fax: 01565 650264
e-mail: courses@pastest.co.uk web site: www.pastest.co.uk